D1038632

Physiotherapy in Occupational Health

Physiotherapy in Occupational Health

Management, Prevention and Health
Promotion in the Work Place

Edited by

Barbara Richardson MSc(London), MCSP, Cert.OH,
Cert.Ed, Dip.TP *Lecturer, School of Occupational Therapy and
Physiotherapy, University of East Anglia, Norfolk, UK*

and

Alfreda Eastlake MCSP, Cert.OH, Grad.Dip.Phys.
Physiotherapist in Charge, Vauxhall Motors Ltd, Luton, UK

With a Foreword by **J. D. G. Troup** DSc(Med), PhD, M(FOM)RCP, FErgS

*Ex-President, Association of Chartered Physiotherapists in Occupational Health;
ex-Consultant and Visiting Professor, Institute of Occupational Health, Helsinki, Finland;
Honorary Senior Research Fellow, Department of Orthopaedic Surgery,
University of Aberdeen, UK*

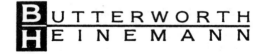

Butterworth-Heinemann Ltd
Linacre House, Jordan Hill, Oxford OX2 8DP

A member of the Reed Elsevier group

OXFORD   LONDON   BOSTON
MUNICH   NEW DELHI   SINGAPORE   SYDNEY
TOKYO   TORONTO   WELLINGTON

First published 1994

© Butterworth-Heinemann Ltd, 1994

All rights reserved. No part of this publication may be reproduced
in any material form (including photocopying or storing in any medium
by electronic means and whether or not transiently or incidentally
to some other use of this publication) without the written permission
of the copyright holder except in accordance with the provisions of
the Copyright, Designs and Patents Act 1988 or under the terms
of a licence issued by the Copyright Licensing Agency Ltd,
90 Tottenham Court Road, London, England W1P 9HE.
Applications for the copyright holder's written permission
to reproduce any part of this publication should
be addressed to the publishers

British Library Cataloguing in Publication Data

RM701
.P494
1994

Richardson, Barbara
Physiotherapy in Occupational Health:
Management, Prevention and Health
Promotion in the Work Place
I. Title II. Eastlake, Alfreda
615.82

ISBN 0 7506 0965 6

Library of Congress Cataloguing in Publication Data

Physiotherapy in occupational health: management, prevention, and health pro-
motion in the work place/edited by B. Richardson and A. Eastlake
p.   cm.
Includes bibliographical references and index
ISBN 0 7506 0965 6
1. Physical therapy.   2. Occupational health services.
I. Richardson, B. (Barbara)   II. Eastlake, A. (Alfreda)
[DNLM: 1. Occupational Health Services – organization & administration.   2.
Physical Therapy.   3. Occupational Health.   4. Occupational Diseases – preven-
tion and control.   5. Health Promotion.   6. Workplace.   WA 412 P578]
RM701.P494
615.8'2–dc20
                                                                94–14343
                                                                CIP

Photoset in 11/12 pt Linotron Palatino by
Wilmaset Ltd, Birkenhead, Wirral
Printed in Great Britain by
Biddles Ltd, Guildford and Kings Lynn

Contents

PUR 9/2/96
DBCW - Acy 6434

JUN 12 1996

Contents

JUN 13 1936

List of contributors

Jeffrey D. Boyling MSc, BPhty, MCSP, MErgS
Director, Jeffrey Boyling Associates, Chartered Physiotherapists and Ergonomists, London, UK

Kate S. Crocker MCSP, Grad.Dip.Phys., Cert.OH
Occupational Health Physiotherapist, A.E.A. Technology, Dorchester, UK

Alfreda Eastlake MCSP, Cert,OH, Grad.Dip.Phys.
Physiotherapist in Charge, Vauxhall Motors Ltd, Luton, UK

Elizabeth A. Edwards BA, Grad.IPM
Personnel Co-ordinator, Vauxhall Motors Ltd, Luton, UK

Joan C. Gabbett Grad.Dip.Phys., MCSP, ONC, Cert.OH, Cert.Ed.
Adviser in Back Care, Kingston & St. George's NHS College of Health Studies, UK

Sheila S. Kitchen MSc, MCSP, Dip.TP
Lecturer, Course Co-ordinator (MSc), Kings College, London, UK

Nancy M. Laurenson BSc, MSc
Exercise Physiologist, British Association of Sport and Medicine, National Sports Medicine Institute, London, UK

David R. Leitch MD, PhD, FRCP, FFOM
Chief Medical Officer, Rolls-Royce plc, Derby, UK

Penny A. Lendon Grad.Dip.Phys., MSCP, SRP, Cert.OH
Consultant Physiotherapist in Occupational Health, Newark, UK

Christopher Norris MSc, CBA, MCSP, SRP, Cert.OH
Director of Norris Associates, Chartered Physiotherapists; Visiting Lecturer to Manchester Metropolitan University at Alsager and London Hospital Medical School, UK

Gillian M. Oldham MCSP, SRP
Occupational Health Physiotherapist, Ciba Geigy plc and Previously with Beechams Pharmaceuticals plc

Stephen T. Pheasant MA, MSc, PhD, FErg.S
Consulting Ergonomist; Associate Professor of Clinical Ergonomics at the British School of Osteopathy; Honorary Consultant at the Robens Institute of Health and Safety, Surrey University; Honorary Lecturer in Ergonomics, University College London, UK

Barbara Richardson MSc (London), MCSP, Cert. OH, Cert. Ed, Dip. TP
Lecturer in Physiotherapy, School of Occupational Therapy and Physiotherapy, University of East Anglia, Norwich, UK

Foreword

The role of the physiotherapist in treating the patient is familiar and greatly valued. But physiotherapists in occupational health go much further. They have unrivalled opportunities for applying preventive measures and they make major contributions to industry and its management. Their potential is, even so, relatively untapped.

The need for physiotherapy in occupational health today can be seen against a background in which the proportion of safety staff for the populations at risk has been falling; in which the number of HSE enforcement officers has dwindled; and in which uncertainties continue to bedevil the National Health Service. Yet against this background the number of physiotherapists in occupational health is on the increase. They have grown in authority as their training and experience have developed, one of the new ingredients in their curriculum being ergonomics.

This new book is particularly welcome. It is comprehensive. It presents a clear picture of the role of occupational health physiotherapists and their place in the management structure of industry; and presents wholly realistic models for the complex aetiology of many of the disorders and ergonomic injuries which have to be prevented and treated.

It gives me great pleasure to recommend *Physiotherapy in Occupational Health* and to wish success to this and all subsequent editions.

J.D.G. Troup

Ex-President, Association of Chartered Physiotherapists in Occupational Health;
ex-Consultant and Visiting Professor, Institute of Occupational Health,
Helsinki, Finland;
Honorary Senior Research Fellow, Department of Orthopaedic Surgery,
University of Aberdeen, UK

Preface

Physiotherapists undertake a wide range of activities which help to restore, maintain and improve the health and physical function of individuals. Carrying these out within the workplace context provides a rewarding focus for the development of expertise and specialization of skills.

Physiotherapists have been working in industry for many years and their numbers are increasing with the development of occupational health services in industry and with the introduction of occupational health departments in hospitals. Physiotherapy services are integral to the healthcare team and can play a significant part, not only in the treatment process but in helping to promote healthy lifestyles which enable people to work to their full potential. This is likely to lead to more job satisfaction and work productivity, and benefits the employer and the employee.

We have worked together for some years in promoting physiotherapy practice in the expanding field of occupational health and have been involved in the development of a postgraduate course for physiotherapists in the field, run under the auspices of the Association of Chartered Physiotherapists in Occupational Health. This book is intended to provide, in a single text, an overall view of the aspects of good occupational health practice which we believe to be pertinent to physiotherapy. It is aimed primarily at physiotherapists with 2 or 3 years' experience who have just started or who are thinking of working in occupational health, but the principles of practice will be of interest to many other physiotherapists for wider application. We hope that it may also assist other health care professionals, as well as managers and safety officers, to appreciate the breadth and depth of the contribution physiotherapy can make to occupational health.

We express our thanks to the contributors. They have been

chosen carefully for their knowledge and experience in their particular subject in order to present the applied and theoretical base of expertise which underpins occupational health physiotherapy. They have all been instrumental in furthering the development of good occupational health practice and generous in sharing their expertise with others. In addition, we acknowledge the many others who have encouraged and supported us in the production of this book and, in particular, Tim Brown, of Butterworth-Heinemann for his guidance and help.

Barbara Richardson
Alfreda Eastlake

Chapter 1

Occupational medicine

David R. Leitch
Penny A. Lendon

History and philosophy

Physicians have taken an interest in diseases associated with occupations since before the sixteenth century. In Europe, doctors such as Agricola and Paracelsus described and even correctly identified the cause of chest diseases in miners. The father of occupational medicine is considered to be Bernadino Ramazzini (1633–1714) who was Professor of Medicine at Padua and Modena. In his book *De Morbis Artifactum Diatriba* (1700), he wrote: 'Medicine like jurisprudence, should make a contribution to the well-being of workers and see to it that so far as possible, they should exercise their callings without harm'. That and many other of his observations remain just as true today.

In Britain, Thomas Percival (1744–1804) was charged with investigating 'factory fever' in Manchester factories. His report to the Manchester Health Board described not only the typhus outbreaks but also the hours and conditions of work of the young employees. Sir Robert Peel (the elder) took up Percival's suggestion of a law to improve conditions. The 'Health and Morals of Apprentices Act 1802' was the beginning of the history of UK health and safety legislation.

If one were to give the sobriquet 'father of British occupational medicine', it would be to the Leeds physician Charles Turner Thackrah (1795–1833). He wrote the book *The*

Effects of the Principal Arts, Trades and Professions of the Civic States and Habits of Living on Health and Longevity (Thackrah, 1831). His work was a stimulus and guide to parliamentary industrial reformers. In it he propounded the concept of industrial health, based on prevention of disease, and the promotion and conservation of health, and physical, mental and moral well-being. While many of his observations on practice remained valid until recent years, there is one which is fortunately of diminishing relevance, namely that: 'The work people are less thought of than the machinery: the latter is frequently examined to ascertain its capabilities – the former scarcely ever'.

Even as modern employers progressively come to limit hazardous exposure, and with today's heavy reliance on service industries of low personal risk, Thackrah still had an appropriate comment: '. . . a master can, a master ought to interfere. He has a right to inquire into the way in which his men spend their evenings, because on this depends their future usefulness to himself'. This view is one which Ministers of Health would support as *Health of the Nation* (Secretary of State, 1991) is pushed forward.

In 1830 a Leeds surgeon, Robert Baker, advised a concerned employer to appoint a doctor to visit his factory daily and observe the effects of work on children's health. He himself later became a factory inspector.

These early doctors and altruistic employers, and politicians, laid the groundwork for occupational medicine. They looked at the effect of work and conditions of work on health, and also the effect of health on the ability to work. Also the concept of health promotion is not new. Prevention of disease appears to have been the moving force in early days. It is curious that in the 1990s many employers seem almost more sympathetic to a treatment service than a preventive service, when historically treatment was quite a late concept. J. & J. Colman of Norwich are believed to have been the first to employ an industrial nurse, one Philippa Flowerday in 1878, albeit with a wider remit than just the workers. In following years the Quaker companies of Cadbury Brothers Ltd. and J. S. Fry & Sons Ltd. set up occupational health services.

Many would consider that epidemiology was a late addition to occupational health. Edward Greenhow, however, who lectured in public health at St Thomas's Hospital in the late nineteenth century, reviewed unpublished records in the Registrar General's Office. Through follow-up he showed that the high mortality from pulmonary disease arising from work was due to dust and fumes. As a consequence the Factory Inspectorate forced an improvement in ventilation.

This brief history of occupational health outlines the background and basis of modern occupational health services. Although an advanced first aid treatment service is, from an industrial employer's viewpoint, the cornerstone, the main activities are about safeguarding the health of employees. First, this is to ensure that the worker and the job are compatible, and second, that the hazards inherent in the job do not adversely affect the worker. These objectives are achieved through a combination of health screening specific to job requirements, advice to employees and management, and health surveillance for the adverse effects of work. All these activities will include a range of general and specific health education.

Occupational health team

The occupational health team can be made up of all the disciplines of health care. It commonly operates within a bigger multidisciplinary group encompassing the three components of health, safety and the environment. The interplay between the three components can be understood if they are regarded as parts of a continuum. Fitness for the job is the start, moving through the physical, ergonomic, psychological and chemical risks and the avoidance of injury, to the removal of hazardous substances from the workers' environment, to the outside world. The broad theme of health runs through all of these.

In large businesses the senior health, safety and environment professional is often the Chief Medical Officer, who in an ideal situation will report to the chief executive or to a director close to the chief executive. The personnel director is often the nominated director. In smaller organizations any of the usual professionals including safety managers, may be the manager of the occupational health department.

Most full-time occupational physicians will be qualified in the field and be Members of the Faculty of Occupational Medicine. Part-time physicians may also have some level of training if not actual qualifications. They may be full-time occupational physicians providing a service, or general practitioners. A growing number of nurses have the new Occupational Health Nursing Diploma and many others have the earlier Certificate. The pattern of employment is varied and in recent years there has been growth in the contract provision of occupational health services. This is driven by businesses reducing the numbers they directly employ to those who make up the core business rather than those who service it. The pattern is widely followed in catering, cleaning and security.

Few companies employ toxicologists or ergonomists directly and it is into the latter role that physiotherapists can be extended. Experienced doctors and nurses will have some knowledge in ergonomics. However, physiotherapists can, with additional training, greatly increase the range and quality of ergonomic advice as a straight extension from the more usual treatment activity. A further group, the occupational hygienists, who investigate and advise on physical, chemical and other hazards, also have some knowledge of ergonomics. With such a wide range of health and safety specialists, collaboration between them is an essential part of teamwork. To avoid conflicting advice being given to managers it is important that appropriate lines of communication are established.

Some companies also employ either directly or indirectly the services of dentists, optometrists and chiropodists.

Why have an occupational health department?

Altruism and moral obligation are very relevant when employers have occupational health services but, as with all health and safety, a major element must be loss control. With that in mind it is then sensible to be able to analyse the work of the department so that the cost of provision can be compared with the benefits gained. There is no doubt that the presence of a physiotherapist in the occupational health team is invaluable in a clinical, preventive and educational role. The gain one would expect would outweigh the cost by a factor of four.

In fact there is no legislative requirement for employers to have occupational health services. They must, however, make provision for first aid. If they have processes which could cause ill health through physical, chemical or other means, and the problems caused could be detected by health surveillance, then they must provide appropriate health surveillance. There are also statutory requirements related to ionizing radiation, lead and asbestos exposure, for which the Health and Safety Executive (HSE) nominates appointed doctors to carry out both screening and surveillance; the results are reported to the HSE.

Employers could meet their legal obligations by simply buying in the services when required. This, however, must be less effective than having them provided by permanently employed people with a detailed knowledge of the processes, the business and the people. A major contribution to loss control in injury and disease under common law stems not from screening and surveillance, but from all the associated activity carried out by occupational health professionals.

Although it is said that occupational health services in general contribute to reduced absence from work, there seems to be a dearth of published evidence. There is little hard evidence for putative material gains resulting from an occupational health service, and no evidence for the claimed soft gains such as improved employee morale and well-being. Clearly, however, many larger employers seem prepared to rely on intuition. This is supported by the fact that many employees with chronic musculoskeletal prob-lems state that direct access to physiotherapy at their place of work does encourage them to remain at work and seek treatment, rather than stay at home awaiting resolution or NHS treatment.

Functions of an occupational health department

The general trend within industry towards trying to achieve better management and employee involvement goes under a variety of titles. Perhaps the best known is Total Quality Management. This has led companies to seek accreditation for their management systems under British Standard 5750 or International Standards Organization 9000 (British Standards Institute, 1987a and b). Inevitably, this has influenced the function of occupational health, even in some cases to the extent that occupational health services have successfully sought accreditation independently from their owning company. Services which take this analytical management approach to their work usually seem to benefit from achieving a clear idea of what are their objectives. Consequently, they are in a better position to gain management support for their continuing existence and aspirations for improvement. It is useful to consider the task in terms of 'outputs', which are the major functions, supported by processes and detailed activities through which the functions are fulfilled.

Major outputs

There are three major outputs, beginning with assessment. These cover the spectrum from potential occupational health hazards, to individual health problems which may affect an employee's ability to work, or may arise because of work. Second, as a result of assessments and interpretation of legislation, advice on the control of hazards can be given to employees and managers. This extends to advice on all aspects of individual employment. The third major output is the provision of services to monitor the health of those exposed to conditions potentially hazardous to health, and a first-aid, general treatment and counselling service.

Processes and activities

There are several activities enabling an occupational health department to identify and assess potential health hazards and factors which are adversely affecting health or performance.

The work of occupational health professionals is never confined to the department or carried out in isolation. Proactive and reactive health and safety inspections, surveys and audits carried out in collaboration with safety and hygiene professionals should be routine. Assessments may be in response to complaints by employees made to their management, or directly to the department. Informed managers may request assessments of suspected problems or situations, where they have recognized deterioration in performance, attendance or quality.

Good record keeping of surgery attendances and treatment patterns, together with analysis of sickness absence patterns will identify acute issues which trigger investigation. Similarly, physiotherapists may recognize a series of similar complaints from one area and be prompted to investigate further. Long-term issues may be identifiable through epidemiological studies of mortality, ill-health early retirement or medical redeployment. For instance, injury records will probably show that manual handling is the major contributor to injury, but that most are hand injuries.

Much work is not in response to identified problems, but is preventive in that hazards are reviewed and exposures monitored, to ensure that risks to health are avoided. Clearly this is a multidisciplinary activity which, in the design and operation of workstations and the ergonomic assessment of systems of work, is amenable to a physiotherapy input. Routine work includes the review of materials and processes to be introduced or in use, and the review and measurement of physical factors such as heat, light, noise and vibration. On occasion, original research work may be undertaken to investigate new health and safety issues and the means by which their effects may be assessed, controlled or eliminated.

Prevention of exposure to risk has many inputs, but all are directed at educating employees and managers. Detailed discussions with managers and engineers are aimed at seeking cost-effective ways to eliminate or control risks.

Health surveillance

Frequently, adequate control of exposure to risk cannot be guaranteed. Where this situation exists, there will be a health surveillance programme if the health effects are detectable. This may extend from the commonplace noise, hand-arm vibration, skin or pulmonary surveillance, to include watching for upper limb disorders in the many potentially at-risk jobs. Most surveillance is carried out by occupational health nurses, but where the issue is musculoskeletal a physiotherapy assessment of identified problems is relevant.

Health screening

Entry to employment is often contingent on being assessed fit to work. In practice, no-one should be submitted to pre-employment medical screening until they have survived the employer's selection procedure for suitability.

The range of approaches is wide. Many companies pay for general practitioners to carry out the examination. Commonly, the medical examination is about fitness to join the pension fund and investigation reveals that no guidance is given to the doctors on the nature of the prospective employee's work. In companies with occupational health departments the trend is to a questionnaire designed to establish the past occupational history, key points of medical history and issues relevant to the job. It is quite usual for these to be reviewed by the occupational health nurses who then carry out a limited physical examination. Perhaps because it is fashionable more than because employers have seen a direct benefit, aspects of lifestyle are enquired into. This gives the opportunity for health counselling. In order for nurses to manage such an approach, they need clear guidance on what are the acceptable findings and what should be referred for medical officer review. While common sense dictates most of the criteria, there are jobs for which quite detailed knowledge is required in order to make a valid judgement. A previous history of recurrent or severe musculoskeletal complaints, especially spinal problems, may well warrant a detailed assessment by a physiotherapist as to the suitability of a prospective employee for a particular job.

Specific standards will be set and in their setting may have received physiotherapy input. Fork-lift truck drivers, overhead crane drivers and workers requiring access to confined spaces would, as examples, need some study of the job requirements so that an appropriate standard could be set.

The primary purpose of the pre-employment medical is to ensure that the job and the person are compatible. Therefore, people with disabilities will normally be assessed by a medical officer. The outcome of such an assessment should be advice to the potential employee and management on how best to organize the job. This may include the marshalling of internal and external resources (Department of Employment) to modified tools, workstations or access. Advice from the occupational health department may lead to quite extensive modifications of job. Much of this can, and does, involve nurses and physiotherapists.

During the course of employment, employers may require confirmation of continuing fitness for the job. Emergency team members and overhead crane operators are just two examples of jobs requiring a reasonable degree of musculo-skeletal and cardiovascular fitness. Although occupational health nurses will carry out much of such screening, specific detailed assessments may be directed to the physiotherapy department. As it would be unreasonable simply to make the declaration of unfit in remediable situations, the physiotherapy department may be involved in the design of advice and fitness training packages for employees.

Treatment

A fundamental activity will always be the first aid and emergency treatment service. Analysis showed that in one large occupational health department, only a quarter of occupational health nurse time was related to the full range of clinical treatment, review and support. Of this, a third was related to injury at work. Continuing treatments initiated by the NHS were normal, but contributed little to the workload.

Carrying out a similar analysis on physiotherapy department work produces a very different picture. In a large company referrals come from many different sources, but generally around 70% of referrals for treatment come from the NHS (GPs, consultants or hospital physiotherapists). Of back problems seen, only about 12% are directly associated with a work injury, although undoubtedly many are exacerbated by the nature of the work. In the younger population, sports injuries are prominent. Lower limb and spinal problems arising from all kinds of injury each contribute approximately 35% of cases. In recent years there has been an increase in the frequency of upper limb problems associated with posture and repetitive types of job.

In the treatment context, physiotherapy departments contribute largely to conditions which have little to do with work. However, if not treated at work, the conditions would certainly cause varying amounts of time away from work, either for treatment or simply because general practitioners would continue to provide certificates.

Rehabilitation

One role of an occupational health department is to be the interface between the Company and employees' medical advisers. A key element of this is to minimize absence due to sickness by encouraging the earlier return of the long-term sick. To do this successfully requires an integrated approach involving choices and combinations of initial part-time work, continuing treatment at work, rehabilitation programmes and modifications of work. The latter may lead to redeployment and retraining to do entirely different work. When financial pressures are tight and in smaller companies, redeployment and protracted rehabilitation may prove very difficult. Managers become understandably less tolerant of markedly reduced performance, and some employees can feel guilty at the burden being carried by colleagues.

When employees with disabilities or with chronic medical conditions are successfully placed or rehabilitated into work, an essential part of their continuing support is regular review. Review will ensure that neither deterioration of the condition nor changes in the job reach a point where employee and job are no longer compatible. In practice, review will usually be carried out by nurses, but may lead to requests for either employee or workplace assessment by a physiotherapist.

For many years there has been a quota system in operation to encourage employers to employ registered disabled persons. This included occupations reserved for such people. The quota is 3% of employees. In practice, few if any private employers have ever been able to reach this level and so have to seek dispensation from the Department of Employment. At first sight this suggests a lack of effort, but there are two relevant factors which give an opposite view. Firstly, people who are only moderately disabled will often prefer not to be registered as they see no practical benefit. Secondly, analysis of workforces shows that up to 8% of employees who are in regular work have medical conditions which meet the criteria for registration as a disabled person. Obviously the quota system serves little purpose in the real world.

Being registered does have one advantage in that it opens access to grants to modify workstations and their access, where this will enable an employer to take on or retain someone who becomes disabled.

Ill-health early retirement

It is inevitable that with life's injuries and ills, some employees will reach a condition where the company can no longer find them useful work, or they are simply unable to work. At this point it should be remembered that companies exist to make money and not to provide charitable refuge. There are limited facilities for sheltered placement but in prosperous times managers tend to be fairly tolerant.

Companies have a variety of routes for terminating employment for medical reasons. The financial consequences of such termination depend on the rules of the pension fund and the company. Some pension funds require a minimum duration of membership before they will pay benefits: this can be as long as 5 years. The pension rules vary between the most severe which will only pay a benefit for total disability, which means exactly that; the employee is unlikely ever to work again. Others have a lesser category sometimes classed as on 'medical grounds,' for which they will pay a smaller benefit than total disability. Medical grounds means various things. It can be as open as allowing retirement on the basis that the employee is no longer able to do the job for which he/she is employed and there is no other economically comparable job available. It acknowledges that the employee might be able to work for another employer even in a full-time capacity. The worst case is where an employee is simply dismissed on the grounds of incapability.

Assessments for ill-health early retirement are usually carried out by company medical officers who, as necessary, seek opinions from general practitioners and specialists. The rules of assessment are fairly simple:

1. Is there a genuine performance or attendance problem?
2. Is the problem the result of a medical problem, be it physical or mental?
3. Is the problem for all practical purposes likely to be permanent?

Three affirmative answers to these questions then lead to the process of grading severity. As the two leading causes of ill-health early retirement are circulatory disease and musculo-skeletal disorders, the latter dominating for manual workers, it is possible for physiotherapists to have some input. For the most part this tends to relate to treatment in the period preceding the decision to consider early retirement. What is recorded in the treatment records can influence the final decision. It is important also to remember that employees now have the right to see their clinical records.

Patterns of work and their effects

Variations of hours of work around the normal working hours have no obvious effects on health. It has never been very clear whether or not rotating shifts which include a night shift have a detrimental effect on health or safety. Every occupational physician has anecdotal evidence that some people are unable to tolerate regular shift work. They become stressed through being unable to establish a proper sleep pattern. This manifests itself in digestive disorders, possibly cardiovascular disorders and various stress reactions. Many general practitioners seem to believe intuitively that shift work must be bad for you.

Shift work is not going to go away, therefore it is necessary to establish what are the least disruptive patterns. These appear to be three shifts rotating forwards, i.e. morning to afternoon to night. Mostly, night shifts are around 8–10 hour. Some companies successfully work 12-hour shifts with breaks of several days between rotations. These, if introduced carefully, are well accepted as they pay well and give substantial periods of time off. Although shifts as such have never really been labelled as a cause of diminished safety, clearly long shifts will lead to fatigue with an obvious attendant risk, but this applies equally to overtime.

Production line work, be it in the pottery business or in car manufacture, is inevitably paced; this removes all control from employees. Low control and high demand, quite apart from the physical demands, are significant factors in causing stress. It is encumbent on occupational health staff who may be called on to advise on aspects of work planning and design, to understand the effects of paced work and the need for rest periods. Some newly-located production line businesses have recruited young people, and have achieved a tremendous pace of physical work. They are discovering that even fit youngsters can wear out and inevitably they grow older and less resilient. It may be that for some jobs employees actually need specifically-designed physical training to prepare them, and also daily warm-up exercises before starting work, to prevent injury.

Discussion of stress is fashionable, yet the problem is real. It has always been around but the nature has changed. In the early industrial days it arose because of enduring poverty, threat to physical safety and the public health problems, largely of infectious diseases. Nowadays its causes are not about these threats to one's very existence, but are more psychological, relating to aspects of control over one's life. It is still commonly thought that stress is an exclusively executive disorder. Nothing could be further from the truth in that many lowly-placed employees experience severe stress for many reasons, some of which are attributable to work. There is a wide understanding of the causes of stress at work and how organizations need to behave in order to prevent it. It is important that companies and managers understand how their structures and behaviour stress the rest of the organization.

Occupational health departments can, in collaboration with managers and personnel departments, run programmes which will educate managers in the prevention and recognition of stress. However, to put it into perspective, every occupational physician will have heard from local doctors that stress is his/her company's disease. In truth, even amongst those considered to be the worst offenders, work either directly or indirectly contributes to well under half of the problems seen. Private life is a major contributor.

Physiotherapists inevitably see people whose problems seem to be without apparent cause. It may well become evident that underlying problems are present. A good ear will identify these. Such cases should always be discussed with doctors and nurses as part of the general 'intelligence gathering' on the health of the organization, which enables occupational health departments to contribute to the well-being of the organization in one of those hard-to-define and unquantifiable ways alluded to earlier.

Health and safety law

Britain has experience of almost two centuries of health and safety law. At present we are experiencing three eras of law concurrently. The Factories Act (1961) and the Offices, Shops and Railway Premises Act (1963), are gradually being phased out under the Health and Safety at Work Act (HSE, 1974). This Act is the enabling Act for all new UK health and safety legislation. All subsequent legislation is in regulations subordinate to this Act. The general principles of health and safety are embodied in Section 2 of the Health and Safety at Work Act which states that so far as is reasonably practicable, employers have general duties to their employees (and others), to ensure their health, safety and welfare at work, through: the provision and maintenance of plant and systems of work that are safe and without risk to health; the safe use, handling, storage and transport of articles and substances; provision of information, instruction, training and supervision; ensuring a safe place of work without risks to health and a similarly safe working environment.

A major change in emphasis came in the Control of Substances Hazardous to Health Regulations (COSHH) (HSE, 1988). These placed a responsibility on employers to carry out a written assessment of risk and to set up a management system demonstrating adequate control of, and protection from, the risks.

The most recent legislation stemmed from the European Commission (EC) general directive and its five daughter directives. The EC is now the prime mover in UK health and safety legislation. The end of 1992 saw six new regulations. Several merely consolidated and refined what already existed, but there were three of significance. The Management of Health and Safety at Work regulations (HSE, 1992a) introduced the principles launched in the COSHH regulations across the whole spectrum of work. This is considered to be the best and most progressive set of regulations since the enabling Act itself. The Manual Handling Regulations (HSE, 1992b) include the same principles and if successfully applied, should help to reduce the major contribution that manual handling makes to injury and ill health. What is considered to be a disproportionately heavy set of regulations in proportion to the risks, are the Display Screen Equipment Regulations (HSE, 1992c). They are an example of union-driven legislation which EC bureaucrats were guilty of failing to research adequately in assessing the true risks to health. However, it must be said that the general guidance is sound, although some of the specific requirements which had to be brought in from the EC directive are impossible to enforce.

Both manual handling and display screen equipment regulations extend the probable demands on physiotherapists to contribute to assessments and advice. In compliance with these regulations, the full scope of a physiotherapist's knowledge can be employed. It is recognized that training in lifting and handling is not the only answer to solving that problem, but that full ergonomic consideration is often more appropriate.

Finally, it should be remembered that everyone in an occupational health department, be they full-time, part-time, contractor or self employed, is subject to the same health and safety regulations as everyone else. Therefore, from COSHH to manual handling, there should be an assessment.

References

British Standards Institute (1987a) *Quality Systems – Guide to Selection and Use*, BS5750 Part 0, Section 0.1 ≡ International Standards Organization 9000, 1987

British Standards Institute (1987b) *Guide to Quality Management and Quality Systems Elements*, BS5750 Part 0, Section 0.2 ≡ International Standards Organization 9004, 1987

Health and Safety Executive (1974) *Health and Safety at Work Act*, HMSO, London

Health and Safety Executive (1988) *Control of Substances Hazardous to Health Regulations*, HMSO, London

Health and Safety Executive (1992a) *The Management of Health and Safety at Work*, HMSO, London

Health and Safety Executive (1992b) *Manual Handling Guidance and Regulations*, HMSO, London

Health and Safety Executive (1992c) *Display Screen Equipment Regulations*, HMSO, London

Secretary of State (1991) *Health of the Nation*. HMSO, London

Thackrah, C. T. (1831) *The Effects of the Principal Arts, Trades and Professions of the Civic States and Habits of Living on Health and Longevity*, reprinted 1989 by Longman Group UK, on behalf of W. H. Smith for the Society of Occupational Medicine

Further reading

Edwards, F. and Taylor, P. (eds) (1988) *Fitness for Work – the Medical Aspects*. Oxford University Press, Oxford

Harrington, J.M. (1978) *Shift Work and Health. A Critical Review of the Literature*, HMSO, London

Harrington, J.M. and Gill, F.S. (eds) (1992) *Occupational Health Pocket Consultant*, Blackwell Scientific Publications, Oxford

Health and Safety Executive (1988) *Essentials of Health and Safety at Work*, HMSO, London

Health and Safety Executive (1990) *Health Aspects of Job Placement and Rehabilitation*, MS23, HMSO, London

Health and Safety Executive (1992) *Your Patients and Their Work*, HMSO, London

Pheasant, S.T. (1991) *Ergonomics, Work and Health*, Macmillan, Basingstoke

Waldron, H.A. (1989) *Occupational Health Practice*, Butterworth-Heinemann, London

Waterhouse, J.M., Folkard, S. and Minor, D.S. (1992) *Shiftwork, Health and Safety. An Overview of the Scientific Literature 1978–1990*, HSE Contract Research Report No. 31/1992, HMSO, London

Chapter 2

History of occupational health physiotherapy in the UK

Alfreda Eastlake

Introduction

To many people the idea of occupational health physiotherapy is a new concept. In fact there have been physiotherapists
working in the industrial setting since 1923, only 3 years after
the Society received its Royal Charter and became the Chartered Society of Massage and Medical Gymnastics.

The number of physiotherapists in industry increased
slowly and the specific interest group, the Association of
Chartered Physiotherapists in Industry (ACPI) was founded
in 1947. Over the years, more industrial departments were
opened and the range of work increased until in 1985 the
name of the Association was changed to the Association of
Chartered Physiotherapists in Occupational Health
(ACPOH). This title incorporated those physiotherapists
working in fields other than industry and thus reflected the
growing interest of the profession in preventive care. Since
then the field has continued to develop and currently (1993)
there are nearly 200 members of the association.

The early years

The first documented firm to employ an industrial physiotherapist was Arthur Guinness, the brewery, in Dublin in
1923 (Hayne, 1977). Only a few firms followed this caring
example until the outbreak of World War II. These included
Pilkington, the glass manufacturers, in Lancashire, Marks
and Spencer, the department store, and Unilever, then soap
manufacturers, in London. The physiotherapists were
employed in order to save time for both the employees and
the firm by providing treatment facilities on site, rather than
at local hospitals.

During the war it was imperative that the fighting forces
and those supporting the war effort at home should remain
fit, and that recovery times from injuries should be as short
as possible. This led to the development of rehabilitation
centres, particularly in the armed forces, where programmes
of graded exercises were found to aid speedy recovery. One
industry of paramount importance was that of coal-mining,
which was also one in which accidents were then common,
and to which conscientious objectors, often not as fit as the
traditional miner, were directed for their war service.
Several centres were established where activities to increase
strength and endurance were performed. These activities
were specifically designed to enable men to cope with the
strenuous and awkward conditions encountered in the coal-
mining industry. Typical of these were centres at Mansfield
in Nottinghamshire and Chester-le-Street in County
Durham.

Following the war, the success of these work-hardening
programmes was recognized and several rehabilitation
centres were founded, often under the auspices of local
hospitals. At these centres patients worked at specific tasks
which produced items for local industry thus helping the
centres to be financially viable. A few industries were large
enough to set up their own centres. Of these Pilkington, in
Lancashire, had their own workshop, and, in 1946, at the
instigation of the local consultant surgeon, L. W. Plewes, a
rehabilitation centre was opened at Vauxhall Motors in
Luton. Using carefully designed machines, this centre

provided tasks that enabled employees to return to their jobs much earlier than they would otherwise have been able, and also to do work that would aid their recovery. At that time, before the welfare state, it also enabled employees to maintain their income. It was run by an engineer and the physiotherapist employed by the firm was very involved with the prescribed activities. Mr Plewes himself visited the centre each week, and closely monitored the patients there.

There are several industrial areas with factories which are individually too small to fund a full medical service. Some have industrial health centres to which the factories may subscribe, and which provide medical, nursing, physiotherapy and other ancillary services. An early example is the Slough Industrial Health Centre, which was founded in 1947 and is still running today. Another method of providing treatment facilities for small firms was that of the Wakefield and District Mobile Physiotherapy Service, which served small industrial units and some rural areas. The physiotherapists used a well-equipped van to visit various locations where treatment could be provided.

As the number of physiotherapists working in industry gradually increased, most working in isolation, there came a need for a forum for them to meet. In 1947, seven industrial physiotherapists founded ACPI; this was one of the first specific interest groups of the Chartered Society of Physiotherapy (CSP) and enabled industrial physiotherapists to meet to exchange ideas, negotiate for better salaries and conditions of service and to discuss how best to develop their role. At this time the physiotherapists in industry were primarily concerned with the treatment of patients, though several were beginning to become interested in analysing the stresses and strains associated with work and in preventing the problems resulting from these strains. This aspect was highlighted at the first World Congress of Physical Therapy (WCPT) in London in 1953, when several continental physiotherapists described work in the field of prevention. The discussions encouraged the UK industrial physiotherapists to develop their skills in analysis and to further their knowledge in the field of ergonomics, 'fitting the task to the man'.

Development

The members of ACPI were anxious to promote their specialized work to the wider physiotherapy profession. To this end the Association published in 1956 a leaflet *Physiotherapy in Industry* (ACPI, 1956). This leaflet explained the work of the physiotherapist in industry and the advantages of having treatment on site, measured both in time saved and, with job-specific rehabilitation, the probability of earlier recovery. At the WCPT congress in Paris in 1959, a meeting of international industrial physiotherapists was held at the instigation of Ernest Tracey, who was then the honorary secretary of ACPI and physiotherapist at the Boots Company in Nottingham. It had been hoped to start an international association of industrial physiotherapists. Sadly this was unsuccessful.

The number of physiotherapists working in industry increased gradually over the years as did their interest in preventive work. ACPI continued to run courses for its members. Some were clinical, to help members keep up with latest treatment methods, others introduced new concepts, particularly those of preventive care. Lectures on the role of the physiotherapist in industry and on manual handling were given at the CSP annual congress in 1962.

As its membership increased so the ACPI became more pro-active in the profession and it became obvious that if members were going to be able to advise firms on preventive measures, they would need postgraduate training in several subjects, among which was ergonomics. An introductory course in ergonomics was held in 1971 in Loughborough. This was followed by week-long courses held in 1972 and 1975 at the Lucas Institute in Birmingham. The main lecturer at both these courses was Professor E. N. Corlett of the Department of Production Engineering at Nottingham University, and a Fellow of The Ergonomics Society. This link with The Ergonomics Society was maintained and further developed when, in 1987, Professor Corlett became President of the Association of Chartered Physiotherapists in Occupational Health (ACPOH) as ACPI had by then become.

The importance of manual handling training in the prevention of back pain remained an integral part of the work of industrial physiotherapists, and has been the subject of many ACPI courses over the years. One which opened the eyes of several members who attended was a course in May 1975 which involved a visit to London docks, where course members had practical experience in handling loads then currently used in the docking industry. These loads were of a size which would now not be considered safe to be lifted manually.

The original leaflet *Physiotherapy in Industry* was much updated and republished in 1974 (ACPI, 1974a) together with another leaflet *Guidelines for Establishing an Industrial Physiotherapy Department* (ACPI, 1974b), which, as its title implies, gave advice on those subjects necessary to consider when setting up a new department. During this period of development in the 1970s, many members of ACPI were active in promoting physiotherapy in industry. Much of the credit for the increase in influence of the Association and its contacts with other organizations, such as the Society of Occupational Health Nurses, must go to Christopher Hayne FCSP, then physiotherapist at John Players, cigarette manufacturers, in Nottingham and honorary Secretary of ACPI.

In the 1970s, industry in general was becoming more aware of the importance of occupational health and safety. This was emphasized by the 1974 Health and Safety at Work Act (Health and Safety Executive, 1974), which superseded the various Factory Acts then in force. It still spells out the legal responsibilities of both the employer and the employee, but is now (1993) being expanded by the European Community's Health and Safety Regulations (Health and Safety Executive, 1992).

Consolidation

ACPI remained active, with a small but stable membership of about 75 members for most of the 1970s. Many of the members were at that time fully occupied with giving treatment, and were not able to broaden their scope by becoming involved with prevention and education. Although the UK had been the first nation to have industrial physiotherapists, they fell behind their Scandinavian colleagues, who rapidly became proactive in the workplace, developing 'pause gymnastic' routines for both factory and office staff (Hayne, 1977) and spending at least half their time on preventive and educative measures. On the other side of the world, Australian physiotherapists also became interested and active in the field of occupational health. As interest in the field of occupational health increased in the UK, more ACPI members extended their role to include aspects of health education and preventive care, such as advising on the choice and proper use of office chairs, assessing fitness for work and lifting and handling training.

As the beneficial effects of exercise in coronary care became more well known, both in preventing attacks and assisting recovery from them, fitness gyms were set up in the workplace. Among the first of these was one at Rank-Xerox, being followed, in 1977, by Marks and Spencer and the Central Electricity Generating Board in London, as well as several others. These first examples were set up partly in order to rehabilitate staff following heart attacks, but also to enable sedentary staff, often executives with very stressful lifestyles, to improve their fitness and thus to help to reduce their stress levels (Lilley, 1983). With an increase in public awareness of the benefits of higher levels of fitness, more companies are providing fitness facilities. Some are 'in-house' and supervised by staff physiotherapists (MacLarty, 1986) or nurses, and others are run by outside organizations.

Despite its small numbers, ACPI worked hard to increase knowledge of the benefits of physiotherapy in the workplace, continuing to provide regular courses and arrange factory visits for its members. These factory visits were especially helpful to members, providing opportunities to see very different industries and thus become aware of a variety of workplaces. As an association it forged and maintained links with other groups with similar interests, such as The Ergonomics Society and the Back Pain Association.

In May 1975, an issue of the Chartered Society of Physiotherapy journal was given over to 'Industrial health'. This contained articles on the role of the industrial physiotherapist and doctor, together with ones on ergonomics, health and safety at work and the industrial nurse's part in health and safety (Slattery, 1975). In later years issues of the journal were also devoted to the subject of 'Lifting' (*Physiotherapy*, 1979), both of patients (animate) and loads (inanimate) and 'Sitting and seating' (*Physiotherapy*, 1984).

Progress into occupational health

In the 1980s interest in preventive care and health education increased among the physiotherapy profession as a whole. Hospitals set up occupational health departments and more people joined ACPI, many of whom were not working in industry. Discussions took place in committee as to how to rationalize these developments, and following the 1984 annual general meeting in Nottingham, a new constitution was drawn up. This was ratified a year later and ACPI became ACPOH. Since then membership has increased steadily, including some private practitioners as well as those working in advisory and consultant categories. The broader interests of the increased membership has led to greater discussion of diverse topics, among which are the problems of manual handling of patients – 'animate' loads.

In September 1988 another issue of the CSP journal was devoted to occupational health. On this occasion there were articles on the physiotherapist's role in assessing fitness for work, prevention and early treatment of musculoskeletal pain, and three articles on various aspects of ergonomics (*Physiotherapy*, 1988). These articles emphasized the mutual benefits to be gained by physiotherapists and ergonomists working together.

Postgraduate education

Although ACPI had run many interesting and varied courses for its members over the years, there was a lack of formal education for those entering the field of occupational health.

In consultation with the CSP, a planning group was formed in 1987 to set up a course, which would be validated by the Society. The planning group comprised Margaret Lilley (Central Electricity Generating Board); Brenda Blair from Shell International (then honorary secretary of ACPOH); Alfreda Eastlake (Vauxhall Motors), immediate past chairman of ACPOH; June Shannon from British Aerospace in Bristol; and Barbara Richardson (née Girling), a physiotherapy teacher from Cambridge with a degree in ergonomics and an interest in physiotherapy in occupational health. The first course 'Physiotherapy practice in occupational health' was granted validation by the CSP and took place from September 1989 to June 1990. Nineteen students enrolled, half of whom were from industry and half from the NHS. The content of the course reflects the broad range of subjects necessary for good occupational health practice, including ergonomics, health education, work physiology, occupational psychology and occupational medicine among the topics studied. The course includes residential periods of theory and development of skills interspersed with workplace visits and an evaluative study. It now runs on a bi-annual basis, and, in line with current educational policies of the CSP, is planned to be integrated into an establishment of higher education.

The future

The work of the early pioneers of physiotherapy in industry has provided an excellent base on which today's practitioners in occupational health can develop successful practice. For example recent legislation (Health and Safety Executive, 1992) requires that manual handling tasks be assessed for risk of injury, and that operators of visual display equipment have suitable workstations. The occupational health physiotherapist is well equipped to recommend measures to fulfil these requirements and to carry out the assessments. The physiotherapy profession as a whole is becoming increasingly pro-active in the field of prevention of musculoskeletal disorders, and this provides practitioners in occupational health with an excellent opportunity to play a leading part in the profession in the consolidation of this aspect of physiotherapy.

References

ACPI (1956) *Physiotherapy in Industry*, CSP, London

ACPI (1974a) *Physiotherapy in Industry*, CSP, London

ACPI (1974b) *Guidelines for Establishing an Industrial Physiotherapy Department*, CSP, London

Hayne, C. R. (1977) The Physiotherapist in Modern Industry 1947–1976. Dissertation for Fellowship of Chartered Society of Physiotherapy, CSP, London

Health and Safety Executive (1974) *Health and Safety at Work Act*, HMSO, London

Health and Safety Executive (1992) *Management of Health and Safety at Work Regulations*, HMSO, London

Lilley, M. (1983) Preventive medicine and the benefit of exercise programmes *Physiotherapy*, **69(1)**, 8

MacLarty, J. (1986) The Fitness Programme at Marks and Spencers *Physiotherapy*, **72(1)**, 54–56

Physiotherapy (1979) Lifting Part 1 and Lifting Part 2 **65(8,9)**

Physiotherapy (1984) Sitting and Seating **69(2)**

Physiotherapy (1988) Occupational Health **74(9)**

Slattery, E. P. (1975) Industrial physiotherapy *Physiotherapy*, **61(5)**, 136

Chapter 3

Role of the physiotherapist in occupational health

Alfreda Eastlake

Introduction

The term occupational health applies to the well-being of people in their working environment, so occupational health departments may exist in many types of workplace: industry; hospitals; homes; shops and offices. Some of these organizations will have large workforces, others only one or two employees. The size of the organization will obviously reflect the size of the occupational health team. An occupational health team may be comprised of staff from many disciplines. It will usually be led by a medical officer and, in addition, will have nurses either with or without occupational health qualifications. There may also be one or more of the following: physiotherapist; radiographer; dentist; chiropodist; safety officer and occupational hygienist. The physiotherapist is very much part of the team, but will almost certainly be working in isolation from any colleagues in the same profession.

The physiotherapist working in occupational health has an important role to play in the efficient productivity of the organization. He or she will have a remit to maintain and improve the working ability of the workforce, thus helping the organization to make a profit, as well as having content and well-motivated staff, working at the peak of efficiency. To achieve this, knowledge and experience of many specialist areas is required in addition to usual physiotherapy skills, such as principles of ergonomics and their application, occupational psychology and work physiology. An understanding of occupational medicine and epidemiology is also necessary.

It is also important to be aware of current and impending legislation, and the implications of these regulations to the workplace and its management; this will necessitate knowledge of how the organization is structured. The occupational health physiotherapist needs to have considerable clinical experience, have confidence in herself, be able to communicate with managers and be persuasive in justifying any proposed recommendation for changes in working practices with understanding of the cost applications involved in implementing these changes. Thus, it can be seen that this will inevitably involve very much more than just clinical treatment; a major part of her role will be to educate and to prevent health problems.

Physiotherapists are trained to take a holistic approach in all their dealings with patients. This entails taking account of the patient's lifestyle, both at work, home and leisure activities. The aim of successful physiotherapeutic treatment is always to restore the patient, both physically and mentally, to as full a life as possible. It is very difficult for the physiotherapist in a hospital outpatient department to be able to visualize the patients' working environments and the tasks performed there. The physiotherapist working in a large organization has an excellent opportunity to observe patients in their own environment, rather than in the strange and, to a patient, sometimes somewhat forbidding, surroundings of an outpatient department.

The pace of modern life has resulted in increased levels of stress-related problems, and the physiotherapist must be aware of this and be alert to the effects of psychological stress on the musculoskeletal system, for example the harassed executive suffering from neck or shoulder pain, or the mother working full-time as well as running a home and suffering from exhaustion.

Traditionally, physiotherapists were employed in industry in order to treat staff injured either at the place of work or away from it. This is still a large proportion of the workload and is efficient in reducing working time lost attending local hospitals (Hayne, 1977) and because treatment can normally be initiated more promptly, many hospital departments being forced to run waiting lists. Because of the occupational health physiotherapist's knowledge of the tasks that the patient is required to perform, treatment can also be aimed specifically at being appropriate for that task, and advice given to the supervisor as to the capability of the patient for light duties or full work. There will probably be many occasions, such as meetings or sporting events, during which the 'patient' will be a 'colleague' and the physiotherapist's traditional role must be adapted accordingly.

The natural progression from treatment and education to prevent recurrence, is towards the prevention of problems that may occur, either in connection with the work activity or because of domestic or sporting activities outside the workplace. Thus, prevention is an important part of the scope of practice of the occupational health physiotherapist.

Treatment

Patients may be referred to the occupational health physiotherapy department by several means: local hospitals; general practitioners; company medical officers; occupational health nurses; supervisors or self-referral. The conditions to be treated will encompass all those seen in any busy outpatient department, but will predominantly be musculoskeletal in origin. It must be remembered that all patients will be of working age, as it is extremely unlikely that the facility would be offered to families of staff, although a few firms may allow retired members of staff to benefit.

Establishments may vary: some will not only allow, but actively encourage, staff who are off sick to attend for treatment, even to the extent of sending transport to bring in those who cannot otherwise attend; other firms will, for various reasons, usually financial, only provide the service to those who are actually at work, even if this work has to be modified. A few firms even have rehabilitation centres, which provide useful and productive work that can be undertaken by those who would otherwise be off sick. In the best of these centres, the tasks to be done can be therapeutic in themselves and be graded and increased in difficulty as the patient's ability, strength and endurance improve. In such centres the physiotherapist is able to provide considerable help in advising which tasks are appropriate for which patient, and on the progression of these tasks. Other firms have systems which will allow staff to return to work on a part-time basis, thus giving them the opportunity to build up stamina over a period of time.

Assessment

As in any form of treatment, assessment of the patient is of prime importance, and in the occupational health setting, may be considered to be even more so than usual. It is necessary to be aware of the specific demands of the task that the patient is expected to perform during the working day, and decide whether he or she is capable of performing it, or if some job modification is desirable and feasible. Thus it can be seen that the scope of practice of the occupational health physiotherapist includes becoming conversant with all the operations of the organization concerned. With this knowledge, treatment can be specifically directed towards those activities necessary to perform the assigned task.

Modifications

When there is the opportunity to have prompt treatment and appropriate work modification available on site, it is often possible for the patient to return to work much earlier. This has obvious benefits to the firm, and also for the patients concerned, who will maintain the work ethic and their self respect, not forgetting their income.

Modifications to the workplace can often be made at no cost

and be very simple, such as arranging a slight change of angle at which a limb is being held, or the use of a different limb. Sometimes rotating tasks more frequently or altering the way a tool is used may, for the worker, make the difference between employment or being at home, off sick. The longer someone is away from work, the more likely it is that they will lose confidence in themselves, and find it difficult to return to work.

Facilities

Treatment facilities required in an occupational health department are the same as those in a hospital outpatient department, although space is likely to be even more restricted than in a hospital. If a new department is to be set up, it should if possible be sited near to the major working area. Cubicles with curtains, and a gym, or at least an area suitable for group exercises are necessary. The physiotherapist should have an office, desk and adequate storage facilities for records. It is most important that there should be somewhere where confidential interviews can be held. The physiotherapist is frequently used as a 'listening ear' and patients must have confidence that any comments made will be absolutely confidential. During interviews of this nature it is sometimes apparent that the cause of the presenting problem is not as simple as it had first seemed. It is of course vital that any information given by the patient goes no further, but the physiotherapist often has to liaise with supervisors and managers, so must be tactful and diplomatic in advising managers as to necessary restrictions on a patient's capability for work.

Techniques

Techniques of treatment will be those normally used in an outpatient department, but possibly with extra emphasis on explanation about the specific condition and the need for home exercises. With sufficient understanding, the patient will be motivated to use natural breaks in the working day as an opportunity to perform a few exercises designed to relieve the tension built up in those muscles used for the task being performed; this is particularly important for those whose work is sedentary. Since patients are receiving treatment during working hours, time must be used constructively and the physiotherapist must be alert to those who may regard a visit to the department as a pleasant alternative to work! Her responsibility is not only to the patient but to the employer of them both.

In the hospital setting it is often necessary to give patients a course of treatment and then discharge them, but in the occupational health setting it is possible to monitor patients for long periods in order to support them through long-term problems. This can be both rewarding and exhausting for the physiotherapist. For the patients, knowing that there is someone with knowledge of their condition, who will advise them should a problem recur or a similar problem arise, is very reassuring and often saves taking time off visiting the general practitioner for minor problems.

In recent years several specialist occupational health physiotherapists have begun to undertake consultancy work. This can take various forms, among which are assessment of the chairs and workstations in an office environment, or the setting up of a manual handling training programme.

Developments

Because most occupational health physiotherapists work in isolation, they can easily miss latest developments in treatment methods, so have a responsibility to keep themselves up to date, by reading and attending courses in relevant subjects. The Association of Chartered Physiotherapists in Occupational Health exists to further communication between its members and to run courses on clinical subjects, as well as on subjects particular to occupational health. The Association also provides a forum for members to exchange experiences and discuss problems; it is recognized in the profession as the voice for those physiotherapists working in occupational health. Two other bodies of particular relevance to the physiotherapist in occupational health are the Ergonomics Society and the Institute of Occupational Safety and Health. (See addresses at end of chapter.)

Records

As in any medical consultation, records must be kept of any treatment and advice given to patients, particularly of any condition which may be work-related in origin. This includes any advice given to the patient or to his supervisor about job modifications. It is becoming more common for physiotherapists to be asked to give evidence in court, or to write reports for legal purposes. For this reason the occupational health physiotherapist must ensure that adequately detailed notes, made at the time of interaction with the patient, are kept. It is possible that these notes may be required as evidence in a court of law, so they must be clear.

The physiotherapist with good knowledge of the workplace will become alerted if several patients come for treatment while working on similar tasks in any one area. This will require a visit to try to discover the origin of these problems, analysis of the cause and likely referral to the works engineer for modification of the task. An example of this type of incident might be several people presenting with wrist problems while doing a task that involves using a mallet. A possible solution would be to ensure that the handle of the mallet be wrapped in shock-absorbing material. In this type of case, the physiotherapist should also be alert to the possibility of 'me-too-ism', particularly where the task in question may be one of the ones least favoured by the workers. A little healthy cynicism can be an advantage, but it is important never to lose sight of the aim of restoring patients to full health, both physically and mentally.

An experienced occupational health physiotherapist will build up a relationship with the workforce and is very likely to find herself used as an advice service. Sportsmen who have injured themselves over the weekend commonly turn up in the department on a Monday morning, for reassurance as much as for treatment. For instance, a man entered in the

London Marathon had a minor hamstring injury 10 days before the race and was, understandably, very worried that his lifetime's ambition might not be achievable. With twice-daily ultrasound, gentle stretching and being persuaded to cut back on his training for a few days, he finished the race in a very respectable time. The day after the race he appeared again in the physiotherapy department complete with his medal and an enormous grin! This sort of opportunity to respond rapidly to a patient's needs is extremely rewarding, and often saves time spent visiting general practitioners, some of whom are not very sympathetic to sportsmen, quite understandably, when they are extremely busy with people who are ill.

Although the occupational health physiotherapist should have broad experience, she cannot be an expert in all fields and must recognize her own limitations, know when to refer a patient on to someone more knowledgeable and not be afraid to admit it when she does not know the answer.

Prevention

Most physiotherapists now working in the occupational health setting are increasingly involved in preventive work, and those working in hospital occupational health departments are likely to be entirely concerned with this, as treatment will probably be performed in the hospital department.

Prospective employees normally have a pre-employment medical examination, and a physiotherapist may well be called to give an opinion as to fitness to perform necessary tasks. This is especially important for those prospective employees who give a history of back pain, but profess to having fully recovered from the former incident. It has been proved (Saunders, 1992) that those who have had one incident of back pain are much more likely to suffer pain than those who have never had a former incident. The employee has a duty to keep himself fit for the task he is expected to do (Health and Safety Executive, 1974), but to be able to do this employees must have adequate training. New employees will undergo an induction course to learn the procedures of the particular firm, the necessary safety precautions and job instruction techniques. The occupational health physiotherapist is very likely to be called in to give advice on general back care and avoidance of upper limb disorders; this may take the form of lectures, preferably combined with practical sessions. Often, these initial courses are followed by refresher courses at later dates. It may be necessary to sign that this instruction has been given (Chartered Society of Physiotherapy, 1992). Working as part of the occupational health team, the physiotherapist may also be required to participate in health education policy. Often, dietary advice will be given as part of treatment, but special campaigns are also common, such as 'No Smoking Day' or 'Look After Your Heart Week'. These campaigns frequently involve the whole occupational health team, and the physiotherapist plays a major role in them.

Manual handling

Manual handling training is also very much part of the NHS scene. It is sometimes forgotten that a hospital functions in the same way as a commercial concern. There are many different tasks to be done and staff need training to perform these safely, efficiently and in a considerate manner. For instance, porters need to be trained in moving inanimate loads, such as gas bottles and filing cabinets, but they also must be skilled in moving patients, and in assisting them to help themselves; these require very different techniques and porters must be familiar with them all. Maintenance men may have been given instruction in back care, but be unable to put this into operation on occasions when, for example, they are working in cramped spaces, such as ducting; they need advice on minimizing the musculoskeletal stress caused by this type of task.

One of the major groups of workers in hospitals is the nursing staff. They are constantly lifting and handling patients, some of whom may be heavy and unable to help themselves. The physiotherapist must be conversant with the types of mechanical aids on the market, and with the application of each. Many hospital beds can be raised or lowered, but often this facility is not used, and sometimes the mechanisms are not properly maintained. The physiotherapist may well find herself to be the one who reports poorly functioning equipment to the maintenance department.

District nurses and other community health workers often have particular problems to overcome, the domestic situation being one where it is not easy to use recommended techniques or equipment. Space is frequently restricted, and hoists and other mechanical aids are not readily available. Staff and family carers working in the home need advice in minimizing hazards, so far as is reasonably practicable. It is often, for reasons of time, not feasible for the physiotherapist to undertake all the training herself. In this case a 'cascade' method is often used; this involves training the trainers. The physiotherapist needs to be a competent teacher well able to get the message across to other people (Chartered Society of Physiotherapy, 1992) and to be aware of the legal implications of training.

As from 1st January 1993 it has been a legal requirement for assessments to be undertaken of manual handling tasks in order to estimate levels of risks and to minimize those risks (European Economic Community, 1992a). The physiotherapist is one of the key members of staff in these assessments and may well be responsible for devising and implementing a programme for these assessments and reducing any risks identified by them. From the same date assessments must be made of the work stations of display screen operators (European Economic Community, 1992b) and staff alerted to the importance of correct positioning of screens and other equipment, proper adjustment of chairs, the importance of taking regular breaks and changes in activity.

The occupational health physiotherapist's advice may sometimes be sought for apparently strange problems. An example of this concerns fork-lift trucks. The suspension on fork-lift truck drivers' seats is minimal, so on uneven floors vibration can be a problem. For females of generous proportions this vibration can be uncomfortable. Safety officers are mostly male and can be somewhat embarrassed to give advice to the opposite gender on the importance of wearing suitable supporting garments. A friendly female physiotherapist is easily able to solve the dilemma!

Fitness centres and company gymnasia

The importance of taking regular exercise and maintaining cardiovascular fitness in order to reduce the risk of heart disease has, over recent years, been well publicized. This has increasingly led to the establishment of company fitness facilities, often in the shape of gymnasia. Occupational health physiotherapists play a major part in persuading management to invest in these facilities, and in planning and setting them up. Some of these are run and supervised for companies by outside agencies specializing in this field. Others are run 'in-house' and are usually staffed by physiotherapists, often with the help of occupational health nurses. For these the physiotherapist must be conversant with fitness testing methods and normal levels of fitness.

Conclusion

The role of the occupational health physiotherapist can be seen as very interesting and varied, with many benefits to staff. It must, however, be recognized that occupational health departments are 'overheads' on firms' budgets, and although the image of a caring employer is an important one, in today's hard-headed world it is important to be able to demonstrate the cost benefits of running such a service. Little research has been done in this area, although one study (Crocker, 1989) shows the reduction in absenteeism resulting from back pain following an education programme. Much more of this kind of research is needed in order to be able, in financial terms, to prove that the cost of providing an occupational physiotherapy service is far outweighed by the benefits obtained. Undertaking this type of research should be a challenge for the occupational physiotherapists of the future.

References

Chartered Society of Physiotherapy (1992) *Moving and Handling*, Fact sheets 9 and 9a, CSP, London

Crocker, K. (1989) Back pain: cost effective management of back pain. *Occupational Health*, **41**, 24–25

European Economic Community (1992a) *Manual Handling*, EC Directive 90/269/EEC, HMSO, London

European Economic Community (1992b) *Display Screen Equipment*, EC Directive 90/270/EEC, HMSO, London

Hayne, C. R. (1977) The physiotherapist in modern industry 1947–1976. Dissertation for fellowship of Chartered Society of Physiotherapists, CSP, London

Health and Safety Executive (1974) *Health and Safety at Work Act*, HMSO, London

Saunders, D. (1992) *For Your Back*, Educational Opportunities, Minneapolis, USA

Useful addresses

Association of Chartered Physiotherapists in Occupational Health, c/o Chartered Society of Physiotherapy, 14 Bedford Row, London WC1R 4ED

Ergonomics Society, Devonshire House, Devonshire Square, Loughborough, Leicestershire LE13 3DW

Institute of Occupational Safety and Health, 222 Uppingham Road, Leicester, LE5 0QG

Chapter 4

Making sense of the organization

Elizabeth A. Edwards

Role of occupational healthcare

In recent years there has been an increased interest in occupational health and welfare. Many employers have become an important source of 'healthcare' for their employees. This 'care' ranges from fitness facilities at the workplace to company-paid private medical insurance. There are many reasons for employers to make use of healthcare professionals and health promotion initiatives. Possible advantages are:

- Healthy employees are likely to be more productive and have less time off work.
- Organizations which look after their employees health and welfare are likely to have a better image, both with their workforce and with the general public.

Research by the Health Promotion Authority for Wales, who studied 200 companies based in Cardiff, Tyne and Wear and Northern Ireland, found that the major factors which prompted health promotion initiatives were legislation, a felt need to improve employee relations by displaying a sense of caring and concern, and staff morale (Sigman, 1992).

In addition, in many organizations there has been a focus on reducing absenteeism. A recent survey by CBI/PerCom (Confederation of British Industry, 1993) showed that the estimated cost of sickness absence in 1992 for UK businesses was £13 billion. An occupational health service can play a key role in supporting and assisting line management in dealing with a subject as emotive as absence.

However, for the health professional this introduces a new set of objectives and demands. The priority in healthcare is usually the patient, but in occupational healthcare there are the needs of the business also to consider. These can sometimes be conflicting and there is an equal, if not greater, responsibility to the organization than to the employee. This prompts the question: 'Why are we here?'. The primary objective of any business is to make money, through creating demand for the product or service and satisfying that demand, with continuing attempts to make the business more efficient. The cost of an occupational health service can run into many thousands of pounds and the business will expect some kind of benefit for its investment. No organization is going to spend money without getting some payback. The occupational health professional will be expected, as are other members of the management team, to show positive outcomes and benefits from the work.

In the context of the organization then, what does this actually mean for the health professional in an occupational setting? The required outcomes or needs of the business will largely depend on the culture and behaviours of the organization. Charles Handy suggested 'six factors' which influence culture and behaviour: size, technology, goals and objectives, the environment and the people (Handy, 1985). So there are a large number of factors which may influence what is actually expected of the health professional in an organization. It may be useful for the occupational physiotherapist to look at where he/she fits into the structure of an organization. What manager does one report to, if any? Which business unit is one part of? These will be influencing factors in identifying the outcomes required by the organization.

Role of personnel

It is often the case that the occupational health service in an organization is part of the personnel department. The changing role of occupational health to a more proactive and preventive service is reflective of the changing role of personnel management in general; it is no longer the acolyte of benevolence of the early 20th century. *Human resource management* is now about developing people and shaping behaviours for future business success. This approach began in the 1980s and is a far more generalist approach than existed previously. It places far greater emphasis on the long-term strategy of the organization than on day-to-day operations. It attempts to link the human resource strategy with that of the whole business far more closely than in the past. In the past, personnel management made the assumption that the people it was attempting to motivate and conciliate were a group of potentially uncooperative employees and a large cost towards the organization. Human resource management takes a far more proactive and supportive view, allowing autonomy and encouraging flexibility in the workplace. These changes could considerably influence the role of the occupational health service in an organization.

Another recent influence on the culture of organizations has been the introduction of *total quality management*. The concept of quality management is no longer something that simply relates to the quality of the product or service that a company produces. It is a far more rounded concept, taking into account the behaviours of people in the organization. These concepts (many organizations have different titles for their version of total quality management) emphasize the importance of attitude, commitment, teamwork and enthusiasm for continuous improvement. Ultimately, its objective is to improve customer satisfaction, but this does not always directly relate to the external customer. It also refers to the 'internal' customer, the person next along the line who receives the work completed so far, be it a product or even a service. The internal customer concept reflects other modern philosophies such as 'right first time' quality and a customer-focused product.

The focus on people reflects the increased interest in occupational health in the workplace and the return of the 'caring employer'. On first glance it may appear that since the 1920s we have come full circle and returned to the welfare approach of early personnel departments. This approach, however, is linked directly to the move towards human resource management that was discussed earlier.

Motivation to work

The focus on people and human resource management approaches relies on the premise that the motivation to work is not based totally on the financial and economic need for it, but also because people wish to achieve, be recognized, take responsibility and gain promotion, or simply that they enjoy the work itself. Identifying what really motivates people at work has been the project of many psychologists and researchers in the 20th century. Probably the most important work is that of Frederick Herzberg, who is known for his 'motivation–hygiene' theory (Herzberg, 1966). This theory grew out of research into an attitude towards work and work motivation of the qualified, professional employee working within the large organization, although his theories have been validated across a wide variety of enterprises and cultures.

Having asked a number of people what made them feel extremely good and bad about their jobs, Herzberg was able to analyse the responses and identify that the subjects most often mentioned were experiences and factors related to a good feeling about the job, in terms of content. Factors mentioned in connection with bad feeling about the job were most often related to the surroundings. These were categorized as 'content factors' and 'context factors'. Herzberg classified the job content factors as 'satisfiers' and the context factors as 'dissatisfiers'. Five factors stood out as the determinants of job satisfaction:

- *Achievement*: personal satisfaction of completing a job, problem solving and seeing the results of efforts.

- *Recognition*: social esteem that results from successful completion of a difficult task, from both managers and colleagues.
- *Work itself*: degree to which work is intrinsically interesting.
- *Responsibility*: having accountability and ownership for socially and personally significant work.
- *Advancement*: changes in status or promotion within an organization, based on performance factors (rather than service, age, etc.).

Herzberg also identified five main influences of job dissatisfaction, known as 'hygiene factors':

- *Company policy and administration*: how well organized and efficient the Company is and the perception of its culture as desirable.
- *Salary/earnings*: justice of reward – is it comparative both internally and externally?
- *Supervision*: competence of the supervisor.
- *Interpersonal relationships*: relevant and regular discussion with management on job-related and performance issues.
- *Working conditions*: state of the working environment; facilities, safety, etc.

These factors had the potential effect of producing, in employees, attitudes principally of job dissatisfaction. If the hygiene factors were held at a high level, the result was not high motivation, but rather an absence of dissatisfaction. So it appears that motivators relate to an employee's relationship with the task that they actually do, whereas the hygiene factors relate to the employee's relationship with the context. In the past, management has relied heavily on hygiene factors to gain high productivity from their employees, but the total quality management approach is an attempt to develop, enlarge and enrich the job, in line with Herzberg's satisfiers.

Change in an organization

Teamwork

In many organizations, systems have been introduced to support the culture changes and improve the jobs, such as team working. It is necessary for the structures in the organization to reflect the behavioural and attitudinal changes required and formal teamworking has become increasingly popular. Teamwork relies on the view that a team of people working together can operate better than the individuals in isolation. However, it is a system which takes time and requires the team to develop its own identity. Teamwork highlights the need for multiskilling, flexibility and versatility. The concept of teamwork is not unique, but it is becoming far more common in organizations.

Stress factors

Although such systems are necessary, they do present problems in the initial implementation stages for organizations, particularly those making changes on a 'brownfield' site. It is far harder to introduce change into an old organization than it is to bring new working practices on to a greenfield site; this is on top of additional problems created by an ageing workforce and an inability to recruit because of reductions in headcount. Ironically enough, these change processes themselves can be responsible for health problems. The stress caused by change can result in emotional, behavioural and physical responses. The uncertainty that change brings with it needs to be managed well, through constant communications and feedback, with assistance from the occupational health service through stress and health training and support.

A business example

The occupational health service in the 'example' serves a workforce of over 5000 employees. It assembles vehicles for both home and European markets. The even greater competitive threat that it faces over the next 5 years is not something unusual in manufacturing industry. Motor manufacturers in particular have been badly hit by the recession and the introduction of new Japanese plants into the UK provides additional competition. The need to become a leaner and fitter organization is therefore not unique. Many employers will face similar problems during this decade. So, 'health-care', health promotion and preventive health care schemes will be a prominent part of the business plan.

The change in management styles here reflects what has happened in many other organizations. In the past the company was an autocratic organization, largely managing through control. Discipline was an important management tool, but rewarding good behaviours was unusual. In recent years the philosophy has changed and it is now far more people-focused, but it will take time before the behaviours of employees, managers and trade union representatives fully reflect this. It may be difficult to see where the occupational health service can fit into this change, but helping to reinforce 'good' behaviours and providing support can assist in making change.

A manufacturing supervisor offered the following example of the 'bad job', the one nobody wanted to do:

"Before teamwork, employees would make use of the system in order to avoid getting stuck on that job. They realized that following a trip to the surgery, and a little note from the doctor, nurse or physiotherapist, they would ensure that they wouldn't get the 'bad' job. I couldn't ignore what the surgery were telling me. With the introduction of teamwork, this job could be distributed amongst the team, and although no one was happy to be on it, at least they knew that it would not be for long. But why don't we change the job? If we really are committed to people we should be looking at making the jobs fit the people and not the reverse."

This example highlights a number of problems for the occupational health professional in an organization. In the first instance, it is vital that links with the supervisor are maintained from the beginning of treatment and throughout it. They have an understanding and knowledge of their people, and will be able to help in making professional judgements, whilst they require the support of occupational health personnel. One must not be naive in thinking that people will not attempt to fool the occupational physiotherapist into believing they are in great pain. They may even have convinced themselves! It is true to say that problems other than physical ones can often result in physical symptoms; the supervisor may be able to give some guidance as to what these may be. In return, the physiotherapist must be able to offer the supervisor essential information, such as the limitations imposed on the work the patient can do, due to their injury. A certain amount of confidentiality must be maintained with the patient, but usable information must be available to the supervisor. The occupational physiotherapist is part of the same management team as is the supervisor, and is there primarily to provide a support service to management and not to replace the NHS or the patient's GP. More importantly, however, one must recognize the opportunity to make strategic changes which have long-term effects, and not be continually fire-fighting. The role of the occupational physiotherapist will differ depending on whom he/she is working with, and Table 4.1 gives a summary of this.

Therefore, the occupational physiotherapist must be seen as part of the management team: someone who has 'bought' into the business objectives as much as any other manager and with responsibility to help achieve them. Only a successful company can support a successful occupational health service, so it must play a role in meeting the competitive threat. Specifically, this can involve personal treatment for an employee: the identification of appropriate work which will not exaggerate the condition or may even assist recovery. Preventive measures can be taken, through education and training or through putting forward ideas on job design, which ensure injuries do not occur. Ergonomically-designed jobs avoid unnecessary lifting and movement, putting components at the right height and close to the point of assembly, to avoid stretching or bending. In short, a well-designed job avoids wasteful effort, which is of benefit to both employer and employee.

Table 4.1 Roles of the occupational physiotherapist

Objectives		
Short-term	*Mid-term*	*Long-term*
Satisfying the needs of the patient	**Satisfying the needs of the first-line supervisor**	**Satisfying the needs of personnel**
Treatment, resulting in reduction in immediate pain, increased movement	Treatment, resulting in increased work output from employee Advice on poor attendees Advice on dealing with consistent medically-related problems	Treatment, resulting in reduction in absence across the organization Development of training to ensure employees avoid injury Support to manage long-term absence Advice on suitability for medical early retirement

Benefits of an occupational physiotherapist

The benefits for the organization are many. Often employees return to work sooner after injury or illness then they would have otherwise. They know that a suitable job will be identified for them with advice from a professional. Better matching of the employee to the job means that employees will not aggravate their health problems through work. They can also obtain priority treatment during normal working time, on site. Not only does this remove the burden from the state, but it usually reduces the time the employee has to wait for treatment and is far more convenient. The combination of the work itself with the treatment can often speed physical recovery. In addition, professional links can be developed with local GPs and hospital staff in a way that would be impossible for any manager or supervisor. This ensures that local GPs are fully aware of the type of work available to employees, and can often result in employees being signed back to work earlier than would otherwise have been the case.

Managing absence

Earlier, the estimated costs of absenteeism across the UK were briefly mentioned. The costs of absence within an organization, both direct and indirect (such as management time and disruption to production) are vast. However, absence takes many forms and it rarely has a simple solution. Management need specialist advice in order to make business decisions about medical conditions. It may be that an employee has a genuine health complaint, whereby physiotherapy at the workplace will speed up recovery and considerably improve the condition. The role of the occupational health specialist here is clear. There is a faster return to work, by providing regular treatment in-house, but without causing severe disruption to the business, whilst working with the supervisor to identify appropriate work during the rehabilitation period; this satisfies the needs of both the employee and the employer. However, genuine medical complaints are not the only reasons for absence from the workplace. Again, it is important that the occupational physiotherapist understands that the continued pressure on businesses to make improvements will result in people problems. The 'genuineness' of an absence is virtually impossible to define, but supervision can be supported in identifying the root cause of the problem.

Job design

In the longer term, the occupational physiotherapist can help make the design of the jobs relate far more closely to the people than they have in the past. Classic methods of job design, particularly in manufacturing industry, have not always taken into account the needs of those doing the job. There are various reasons why changes are needed. With organizations supporting and promoting total quality management programmes, there must be visible improvements for employees to become genuinely committed to the change. In the past the design of jobs has been very mechanistic, based on the scientific management approach, designed around the turn of the century by Taylor, using stopwatches and timings down to seconds. For those working in jobs where the physical stresses and strains are many, the occupational physiotherapist can help by developing, with supervision and engineers, to plan the work better for the people. Although in the short term this may appear an expensive approach, the cost benefits can, ultimately, be considerable, through reduced absence, hospital and surgery visits and accidents at work. Individually, these can cost organizations many thousands of pounds. For example, in recent months 'repetitive strain injury' (RSI) has been high on the agenda. RSI is a disease that has largely affected employees doing repetitive physical work, such as assembly line workers and keyboard operators. Although this is still a controversial complaint, many would claim that it can be prevented or reduced through better job design. The TUC and Health and Safety Executive made the following recommendations in 1989 (some of which have now been superseded by the new Health and Safety legislation) (ACAS, 1990):

- work organization allowing frequent breaks from the keyboard and a variety of tasks
- training for employees regarding the risks of RSI
- special exercise programmes
- ergonomic design of tools, workstations and equipment.

In addition, as an equal opportunities employer, job design must account for the differences in physical strength between many men and women. It is likely that the changes in legislation introduced through the European Community will strengthen an employee's right to claim direct and indirect discrimination of an employer. Any positive steps to promote fairness and equality could result in large savings in the long term, by avoiding costly tribunal cases.

Health and Safety legislation

The recent changes in Health and Safety legislation from January 1993 also introduced new requirements for employers. These included the need to formally assess risks and establish means of avoiding them and requirements for those using visual display units (VDUs) as a high percentage of their work. The European approach to Health and Safety legislation has been to enforce employers to take a far more preventive approach, and here the occupational physiotherapist can assist. Ensuring that potential physical risks are identified and avoided, be it through training, re-instruction or ergonomic design of work to suit the requirements of the workforce, process and product, can assist an employer in complying with the regulations. It is likely that this proactive approach will become a bigger part of future legislation, and this is a growing opportunity for occupational physiotherapists to have an impact on the organization.

Trade unions and occupational health

The relationship between occupational health professionals and trade unions is a complex one and can lead to a conflict of interest, particularly as regards disclosure of information and medical confidentiality. Depending on their involvement in the organization, trade unions can have an impact on the health and safety policy and, through safety representatives, they often play a part in its implementation. It is important to liaise with trade union representatives to gain their support, or at least their understanding. They may still create conflict, but this is only to be expected. In the past they saw the 'welfare' of employees as a major part of their role, and it is no surprise that they may be cynical about an organization taking a proactive approach to healthcare. They often see these steps by management as a means of undermining or bypassing them. It is true that the development and increased use of human resource management approaches and total quality management strategies has coincided with the decline of trade union power, but it is claimed that this is a consequence and not an objective of these approaches (Marchington and Parker, 1990). It will take time for them to change and recognize that the role of the occupational health professional, although part of the management team, is not a direct threat to their role, nor are they in existence simply to help management dismiss poor attendees. In the booklet *Health & Employment*, the Advisory, Conciliation and Arbitration Service (ACAS) make the point that 'employees and trade union representatives are likely to be sceptical of health initiatives if basic health and safety provisions are not of a good standard. It is therefore vital that organizations have effective health and safety policies and practices on which to base broader health measures' (ACAS, 1990).

The problem of isolation

Teamwork and being part of the management team has been mentioned many times throughout this chapter, but in fact there are specific problems for occupational physiotherapists in the commercial organization. Due to their specialization, they are extremely isolated. They rarely get time to meet with other physiotherapists, whereas in a hospital they would have the opportunity to meet colleagues and exchange information on a professional level. It is important that an effort is made to keep up with new techniques and developments within the world of physiotherapy, but without it distracting from their primary role. Developing links with other occupational physiotherapists, or with a physiotherapy team at a local hospital, may help. Alternatively, they can develop contacts through the Association of Chartered Physiotherapists in Occupational Health.

Conclusion

The occupational physiotherapist in an organization has a difficult role, with employees, trade unions, line management and personnel all making demands. However, with the changes towards more 'people oriented' organizations, through total quality management programmes, human resource management approaches and 'teamwork', the occupational physiotherapist has the opportunity to make a direct contribution to the success of the business as a whole. By developing and implementing preventive policies and involvement in job design, improvements can be made in attendance, injuries at work and the long-term health of employees which ultimately affect quality, cost and efficiency.

There is continued pressure in business to make improvements, and it is necessary for the occupational physiotherapist to be seen to understand these, and to assist in achieving the necessary improvements. This requires an understanding and awareness of business matters not required of physiotherapists employed outside occupational health services. In addition, displaying this commitment to the health and welfare of employees can help with the implementation of change processes. Once employees see management walk like they talk, then they too will make changes in their behaviours. So the occupational physiotherapist can even impact on the long-term behavioural change in organizations, in additional to the short- and mid-term needs that they satisfy.

References

ACAS (1990) *Health & Employment Advisory Booklet 15*, ACAS, London

Confederation of British Industry (1993) CBI/PerCom Survey of Absence from Work – *'Too Much Time Out'*, CBI, Harvester Wheatsheaf, London

Handy, C. (1985) *Understanding Organisations*, Penguin, London

Herzberg, F. (1966) *Work and the Nature of Man*, World Publishing Co., USA

Marchington, M. and Parker, P. (1990) *Changing Patterns of Employee Relations*, CBI, Harvester Wheatsheaf, London

Sigman, A. (1992) The state of corporate healthcare. *Personnel Management*, Feb

Chapter 5

An ergonomic approach to assessment

Barbara Richardson

Introduction

People often adapt themselves to difficult situations at work and accept high levels of effort or discomfort as an inevitable 'part of the job'. But as Pheasant (1991) points out, they may suffer injuries and strains from bad working postures, have less spare capacity to deal with emergencies, have greater probabilities of accidents and greater probabilities of error. Musculoskeletal problems form the basis of the work of both the occupational health and outpatient physiotherapist, and it is becoming increasingly obvious that physiotherapy has a much greater role to play in areas of prevention and education as well as in treatment. Whilst at work each person is an individual with the potential to build up musculoskeletal stress in an individual way and each person will react differently to the same workplace demands. Although the aim is to minimize the stresses that exist in the workplace for each worker there will often of necessity be a need for compromise. There is a professional responsibility to investigate the roots of the problem for each individual patient and to make sure that each person is educated in strategies to prevent recurrence. Recommendations for changes in the workplace should ideally apply to the specific working practice of the individual, but a responsibility also lies in contributing towards programmes of prevention for the benefit of the workforce as a whole.

Musculoskeletal stress

It is now accepted that it is rare for a single dynamic movement to result in a disorder of the musculoskeletal system but rather that the problem is cumulative, building up over days, weeks or months (McKenzie, 1983). Tissues may become stressed gradually by repetition of poor postures or lifting heavy loads and there is often a history of intermittent aching before a full blown problem incapacitates the worker (van Wely, 1970). This can occur as a result of many factors concerning the biomechanics of working postures, such as the angles at which body parts are stressed, the weight or dimensions of the load, or the mechanical leverage which is built up through handling at a distance. Effects of other factors from the immediate or general environment such as working temperature, uneven floors, management pressure to work faster, or peer pressure to do the work in a particular routine, may equally load the musculoskeletal system of the worker and contribute towards an unhealthy level of stress, but are not always considered.

The pathogenesis of musculoskeletal stress involves physiological and psychological factors which contribute to a pattern which is unique to the individual; it does not become manifest in easily detectable signs for the worker, his colleagues or the clinician. There is a further problem in that the wide range of human pain thresholds (Bond, 1979; French, 1992) makes responses to discomfort immensely variable and will influence how and when stress of this nature is reported (Helman, 1986). As a consequence, there is a lack of epidemiological description and this is a major limiting factor in effective control of work-related disorders of the musculoskeletal system, because it precludes a definition of musculoskeletal stress that can produce precise guidelines for its prevention.

Physiotherapy and ergonomics

In preventive practice, the occupational and leisure activities of people are scrutinized closely in order to spot any mismatches between the demands of the work and the capabilities of the individual. Both sides of the question are considered – the person and the job. This is where ergonomics comes in. Ergonomics aims to 'fit the job to the man' (Grandjean, 1988). The discipline of ergonomics is based on the sciences of human behaviour and human capacity, and involves the application of biological and physiological knowledge to technology and work. Essentially, ergonomics takes a person-centred approach to management of problems to try and maximize the relationship between workers and work in order to optimize the well-being and efficiency of the worker. A multidisciplinary collaboration is needed and Singleton (1982) believes the only feasible vehicle for widespread application of this approach is through other disciplines. He emphasizes the style of thinking of the ergonomist which, whether adopted by a doctor, engineer, physiologist (or physiotherapist), encourages a unique interdisciplinary approach which is focused on the person who is working and oriented to work.

Managing the problems which result from poor working practices gives physiotherapists a unique insight into the aetiology of those problems and puts them in a good position to utilize ergonomic principles in attempts to prevent them from occurring. As Corlett and McAtamney (1988) stated: 'Those physiotherapists who have worked with people in the workplace will know how well suited physiotherapy skills and techniques are to the assessment and evaluation of ergonomic factors and to prevention of work-related musculoskeletal disorders'.

Ergonomic approach

The principles and practice of the discipline of ergonomics are based on the study of systems, a system being defined as a 'group of objects with a group of relationships between these objects' (von Bertalanffy, 1950). It is the specific interrelationship of the separate parts of a system which function together that effects the purpose of the system as a whole. For example, a bicycle is a simple system composed of many parts such as pedals and wheels; each has a separate function but when working together they will predictably effect the work of the system of the bicycle. Another part and other interrelationships are added to the system when a human operator sits on it, and another system then exists which is less predictable than the bicycle alone since the capabilities of the worker and the way he applies them are less easy to define (Romiszowski, 1970).

So, in taking a systems view of a problem between workers and work, the discipline of ergonomics is concerned not only with factors of the workplace part of the system, or organization, and its arrangement but also with factors in other parts of the system, such as the environmental control part of the system or the management part of the system. Each will interrelate with the workplace part of the system and the worker part of the system. The whole organization, therefore, is regarded as an interactive sum of its parts which include the worker, his interface with the equipment at work, the immediate environment around him and the organizational environment generally surrounding those.

An ergonomic approach to assessment of work in an organization considers the worker as an integral and interactive part of the system, and his activities in a workplace at any one time are seen to interact or be affected by spheres of activities in other parts of the organization. The aim is to consider if the system best fits the work to the worker and this has to be determined from within the framework of constraints which are present in each individual situation. Constraints could, for example, be imposed by limitations of the equipment provided or of the lack of working space, or equally by limitations of the people concerned, whether management or workers, or the limitations of the type of work involved, such as production-line work.

The ergonomic approach is particularly suited to assessment of risk for musculoskeletal stress of workers because there is no proven causal relationship on which to take direct action, and a build-up of stress may be imposed upon the worker from a number of diverse factors in the organization. In using this approach many more factors are likely to be recognized as potential stressors of the musculoskeletal system of the worker, such as economic and management issues or the psychosocial attributes of the individual. Looking at the organization as a whole can also show how potential problem factors interrelate and compound or diminish each other. For example, a problem in the workplace with a piece of equipment which is considered risky because of the effort required to use it may be compounded or diminished by the level of competence of the maintenance department, or the management practices for correct procedures.

Assessment

The aim of ergonomics is to fit the job to the worker. The aim of an assessment is to identify the factors which may give rise to musculoskeletal stress in the worker. Through careful observation and description of the work activity these factors can become evident, together with their interrelationships, and can give some indication of the best approach for taking preventive measures. The ideal is a work system in which physical risks to the worker are kept low, i.e. will not lead to work-related musculoskeletal stress. The challenge is to discover key risk factors and to eliminate or reduce them through manipulation of the system, by changes in the workplace, the job, the behaviour of the worker or the behaviour of management for example, in order to achieve a safe system of work.

It is obviously necessary to look at the work itself and the workplace in which it is being carried out, and also at the individual worker and the organization (Shackel and Whitfield, 1969). To ensure that the multiplicity of factors that contribute to musculoskeletal stress are investigated in each part of the system, it is helpful to look for physical problems of the situation such as equipment or workspace, behavioural

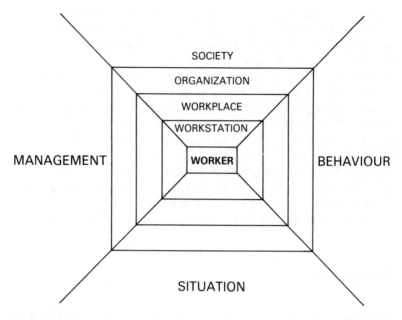

Fig. 5.1 The worker in a system: a model for assessment of risk of musculoskeletal stress.

problems in the way tasks are performed, or interaction between people and influences from others, and managerial problems in the way the job is organized and supervised (Fig. 5.1; see also Girling and Birnbaum, 1988).

A multifactorial assessment made through an ergonomic approach can clearly be carried out in the workplace itself only through an unobtrusive observation of working activities which simply attempts to evaluate the reality of the worker's interface with the work. Use of monitoring devices might weigh the worker down or interfere with performing the task; however, measurements of workers, their equipment or loads can be made as necessary and, if possible, the task itself should be tried by the assessor to determine if an untrained person is able to make the required grip or create the required force, etc. without feeling strain. Workers should also be asked what they think. They usually know very well which parts of their task are stressful even if they do not take steps to change them (Luoparjärvi, 1987). In some working situations it may be acceptable to use videos and photography for later scrutiny, and this is a particularly useful way to capture evidence of a poor working posture or practice. Subsequently, this may provide useful feedback to a worker and could also be a useful tool in solving problems in the workplace.

Junior managers, foremen and safety representatives are likely to be involved with risk assessments to comply with Manual Handling Operations Regulations (Health and Safety Executive, 1992) and often it can be beneficial for assessments to be made by a small working party to give an all-round perspective. This group might also include the occupational health doctor, nurse, health and safety officer, as well as the occupational physiotherapist and any other professional who may be concerned with the health and well-being of the worker in a particular organization.

In any observation of activity in the workplace there must be a sensitive appreciation of possible issues or conflicts between workers, employers and professionals (Horan, 1993). It is important to be seen as being professionally objective and neutral by all parties if further work with a workforce is to be acceptable and credible.

Procedure

Observations from each part of the system form the basis of a risk assessment of work activities and they need to be recorded. Standard forms in the format of checklists can be agreed and produced within an organization (see Health and Safety Executive, 1992; McAtamney and Corlett, 1992; Birnbaum et al., 1993) or observations can be recorded in any way that allows a later scrutiny to be made, e.g. video, tape recorder.

The worker

Assessments should start with the worker. The occupational health physiotherapist will usually have a specific worker in mind; if a patient is part of the workforce with which the physiotherapist is working closely, it will be easy to gain some idea of an individual's physical capabilities or disabilities from medical records or the occupational health doctor prior to the assessment. Other individual characteristics such as size, sex, strength, age and ethnic background should be noted, as well as the individual level of training, skills, and experience. The fitness level of workers is important: the young in particular may be in a more disciplined work routine than they experienced at school, with no idea of how to pace themselves. Personality, motivation, state of health, substance abuse, role in the organization and stage of shift work or time of day may also play a part in contributing to the potential risk of individual work performance.

If the assessment is to be carried out to comply with Manual Handling Operations Regulations (Health and Safety Executive, 1992) it may focus on the task itself, with an average worker in mind who has characteristics based on assumed norms and averages of health, stature and physical dimensions of the population in general. Detailed data of the latter fall within the realms of anthropometry and may be studied in Pheasant (1986), or Grandjean (1988).

The workstation

Assessment should then look at the workstation, a term commonly used to include the worker, the equipment and the work activity. Physical and mental characteristics of the worker should be compared with the dimensions and demands of the equipment, the immediate environment and the task. Good workstation design, which keeps musculoskeletal stress to a minimum, allows the largest and the smallest person to have adequate space clearance to move and perform work with joints at about the midpoint of range, and to adopt postures during the work task which incur minimal biomechanical stresses. The strength and exercise tolerance of the worker should be sufficient to match the demands of the task and psychological stimuli should not be a distraction.

Criteria for acceptable workstation design bear a relationship to each other. Posture will be determined by the relationship between the dimensions of the worker and the dimensions and the conditions of the workplace and the work equipment. Postures of more than 20–30° of neck flexion from the vertical and more than 30° of flexion of the lumbar spine from the vertical should be kept minimal (Nachemson, 1991). The force a worker is capable of exerting will be strongly influenced by posture, in particular the position of the hands and feet, e.g. hands produce less force the further above shoulder level they are required to work. The working posture ultimately taken up will affect or be affected by the visual requirements of the task, e.g. sewing, scanning visual display units, reading notices, etc. The preferred zone for location of visual displays lies between the horizontal line of sight down to an angle of 30°, although it can be extended through another 15° with an acceptable small amount of flexion or extension of the neck (Pheasant, 1986). General visual focusing distance varies with different studies but is thought to be around 500–600 mm (Grandjean, 1988). The focusing requirements of the task and the eye–hand co-ordination required can be crucial and may compromise each other.

Principles for the optimal arrangement of work to keep musculoskeletal stress minimal (Corlett, 1983) concur very much with physiotherapeutic principles. The work should be adequately visible and the worker able to maintain an upright, evenly balanced and forward facing posture, and to adopt several different safe postures without reducing the capability to work. Work should not be performed consistently above the heart and static postures are as stressful as dynamic in compromising the cardiovascular system and hence creating musculoskeletal stress. Standing still should be avoided. Muscular force is best exerted by the largest appropriate muscle groups with the limbs working at 90° to the load and it should be possible to use a variety of muscle groups. Body weight when standing should be carried equally on both feet, with sufficient space to allow weight transference as needed. In sitting, the feet should be supported adequately, and support also given to the task or the hands if necessary to ensure that the wrist, hand and elbow are in alignment. Rest pauses, whether formal or informal, can be crucial to minimizing the build-up of stress; they should be adequate to allow for all loads experienced at work, including environmental and information loads, as well as the length of the work period between successive rest periods. Other factors in the immediate environment, such as protective clothing, may also limit movement and add to the load on the musculature of the worker.

Different types of workstation, e.g. seated, standing, manual handling, have specific areas of concern with regard to potential build-up of musculoskeletal stress and more detail and checklists may be found in Grandjean (1988) and Pheasant (1991).

Task analysis

A task analysis is carried out to ascertain more precisely how stress and fatigue of the musculoskeletal system of the worker may arise. Factors of the task, such as strength required, postures and strategies which are being adopted to carry it out should be noted. A single piece of work may comprise many tasks and it may be necessary to look at each in order to identify problems and to determine the approach to future management of the work and reduction of risk. Moving boxes into a store, for example, may incorporate one task of taking the box from a trolley, another of carrying it through the store and another of putting the box up onto a shelf. Each task should be defined and note made of the duration and frequency of each action and whether it calls for maximum or minimal pressure to be exerted. Critical body measurements for each action, whether the actions are in an awkward direction in relation to the body, and how that may affect the force that can be exerted should also be noted (Galer, 1987).

The workplace

A poor posture or a heavy lift may be acceptable for a few seconds on one occasion, but not if repeated often during a working day, or carried out in an area which is full of obstacles. The task should therefore be viewed within the perspective of the design of the job itself and the hazards which may be present in the workplace, the environment in which the specific work activity is taking place. Stress to the worker may arise as a result of factors such as noise, heat, cold, humidity, draught, ventilation, light, toxins, obstacles, social factors, vibrations, dust, management; in particular: tolerance to heat in the workplace will affect the threshold of fatigue of muscles (Kerslake, 1982); undue noise levels in the workplace can be linked to tensions which may lead to musculoskeletal stress (Jones and Davies, 1982), and lighting has a direct association with musculoskeletal stress since it has a bearing on the posture adopted to perform the task (Boyce, 1982). The way the task relates to the cycle of work, how often it is repeated, the lengths and frequency of the rest breaks, whether it is heavy sustained work, static work or repetitive work and whether there are other loading tasks, may all be significant. Paced work or piece work may have a particular influence on the overall musculoskeletal loading of a worker, as will the hours of work, whether it is shift work and whether the workers rotate through various duties.

The organization

Appraisal of the interaction between workers, or workers and management within the organization can give a clearer understanding of the way the task is related to the whole workload. The authority that is exercised over the way the task is carried out or over the worker carrying out the task and whether rules and procedures are considered necessary, can be very informative. Also of note is how much forward planning of the work takes place to avoid bottlenecks, the procedures for purchasing the equipment used, and whether worker well-being is seen to be important. The latter may be witnessed by adequate provision of aids, equipment and training. Other issues to note in the organization part of the system are the channels used for communication, such as interdepartmental meetings, and how procedures and instructions are generated and disseminated to the work-force. The general feeling or ambience of the workplace can also be pertinent.

Society

Finally, outside influences from society into the work system may be identified and can be of importance with regard to planning any programmes of improvement. For example, regulations such as the Manual Handling Operations Regulations (Health and Safety Executive, 1992), will often make certain aspects of reduction of musculoskeletal stress a priority within the organization, and legislation or the fear of litigation is a significant argument for change. It may also be the case that certain items of equipment are promoted to the organization by high-pressure salesmen and are likely to be chosen because of the marketing skills of the producer rather than the suitability of the equipment for the task concerned. Similarly, items may be cheaper and fulfil specifications but still not be sufficient for safety, e.g. gloves may be of adequate size but have insufficient reinforcement of the palms and fingers.

Clearly, a multifactorial assessment such as this (see Fig. 5.2) can only identify factors which may increase the risk of work-associated problems. However, since the very nature of musculoskeletal stress does not allow for each factor to be proved in isolation, it can be an effective way of becoming aware of patterns of stressors which may not be as obvious in a subjective report from the worker or from a cursory appraisal by a line manager.

Problem lists and action plans

The problems identified in each part of the system are then drawn together into a list. Those identified in the workstation are scrutinized within the perspective of workplace problems, to see if they interact or are constrained by them, and then, in turn, to see if they are regulated by influencing factors noted in the organization. For example, problems of poor job design or lack of attention to environmental factors noted in the workplace may be further substantiated by a lack of information to managers concerning the arrangement of jobs or the attitudes towards worker well-being noted within

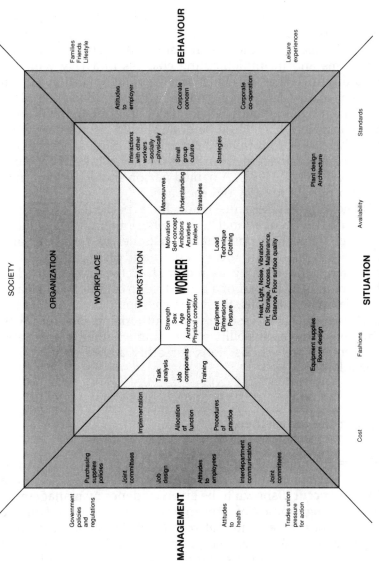

Fig. 5.2 Some areas for investigation in a multifactorial assessment of risk for musculoskeletal stress.

the organization. In this way, a hierarchy of influences can emerge.

The dynamic nature of interrelationships of activities within all areas of the organization should be clearly highlighted and will assist in the identification of routes for solving problems and in implementing changes in a way which is meaningful to the individual organization. An action list can then be made which prioritizes changes to be made according to risks judged as mild, moderate or severe. An idea of the time in which this should be done should also be given and whether the actions involve changing physical aspects of the workplace, management organization or worker behaviour (Birnbaum et al., 1993). A named person should be identified as appropriate to carry out each action.

Following assessments made for a particular worker or patient, the occupational health physiotherapist can make contact with the appropriate personnel to negotiate and initiate any changes in the workplace and carry out individual education and training as required. If the assessment has been requested as part of a procedure to comply with Health and Safety regulations, the action list should be signed, in the presence of the assessor, by the authorizing manager who then has the responsibility of choosing whether to agree and implement the actions, look for other advice or to call in consultants.

Using the assessment

Successful implementation of the concept of risk as a rationale for prevention of musculoskeletal stress is more likely to occur if shown to be given credence by management and if programmes of prevention are implemented in the organization as an integral part of the functioning of that organization. As Spear (1980) pointed out, the 'objective' reality of safety and preventive measures is determined by the individual's 'subjective' model of reality; action is taken according to perception and interpretation of events in the workplace. If workers do not perceive any concern for problems of risk to the musculoskeletal systems of workers in the events occurring around them, then they are unlikely to take any action themselves. Luoparjärvi (1987) suggested that where possible there should be a facility for critical appraisal of the workstation, the job design and working procedures by workers themselves, which can then be seen to be acknowledged and acted upon by management. Workers in the workplace who carry out tasks as part of their work need to be involved in making assessment of those tasks. The person undertaking the job is often the one with the ideas and the experience to describe the difficulties and the areas in need of improvement. In doing so he is also able to define his own objective reality of risk.

A team approach is crucial to realistic measures being taken and acted upon by the workers. This is underlined in recent reports of studies into the feasibility of participative ergonomics which suggest that 'participation is seen as providing the opportunity for real, early and full involvement of the people involved – operators, supervisors – in making decisions about their jobs, systems, workplace and organisation' (Wilson, 1991). Careful consideration should be given to the desirability, both from a financial and sociological point of view, of calling in experts from outside the organization to make risk assessments. At least initially it would seem that there is more to be gained from assessments made within the workforce by working groups which represent a cross-section of the organizational perspectives. The economics and the cost benefits of proposed changes should be better considered, and solutions drawn from such groups on the arrangement of safe systems of work are more likely to be accepted by managers and workers alike. The occupational health physiotherapist should play an active part in their promotion.

References

von Bertalanffy, L. (1950) An outline of general systems theory. *British Journal of Philosophical Science*, **1**, 134–165
Birnbaum, R., Cockcroft, A. and Richardson, B. (1993) *Safer*

Handling of Loads at Work, 2nd edn, Institute of Occupational Ergonomics, University of Nottingham

Bond, M. R. (1979) *Pain, Its Analysis and Treatment*, Churchill Livingstone, Edinburgh

Boyce, P. R. (1982) Vision, light and colour. In *The Body at Work*, Biological Ergonomics (ed. W. T. Singleton), Cambridge University Press, Cambridge

Corlett, E. N. (1983) Analysis and evaluation of working posture. In Ergonomics of Workplace Design (ed. T. O. Kvålseth), Butterworths, London

Corlett, E. N. and McAtamney, L. (1988) Ergonomics in the workplace. *Physiotherapy*, **74**, 475–478

French, S. (1992) The sociology and psychology of pain. In *Physiotherapy, A Psychosocial Approach* (ed. S. French), Butterworth-Heinemann, Oxford

Galer, I. (1987) *Applied Ergonomics Handbook*, Butterworths, London

Grandjean, E. (1988) *Fitting the Task to the Man*. Taylor and Francis, London

Girling, B. and Birnbaum, R. (1988) An ergonomic approach to training for prevention of musculoskeletal stress at work. *Physiotherapy*, **74**, 479–483

Health and Safety Executive (1992) *The Manual Handling Operations Regulations and Guidance on Regulations*, HMSO, London

Helman, C. (1986) *Culture, Health and Illness, An Introduction to Health Professionals*, Wright, Bristol

Horan, S. (1993) Absolute confidentiality – myth or reality. *Occupational Health*, **45**, 16–18

Jones, D. and Davies, D. R. (1982) Hearing and noise. In *The Body at Work*, Biological Ergonomics (ed. W. T. Singleton), Cambridge University Press, Cambridge

Kerslake, D. M. (1982) The effects of climate. In *The Body at Work*, Biological Ergonomics (ed. W. T. Singleton), Cambridge University Press, Cambridge

Luoparjärvi, T. (1987) Workers education. *Ergonomics*, **30**, 305–311

McAtamney, L. and Corlett, E. N. (1992) Ergonomic workplace assessment in a health care context. *Ergonomics*, **35**, 965–978

McKenzie, R. A. (1983) *The Lumbar Spine: Mechanical Diagnosis and Therapy*, Spinal Publications, Waikanae, Wellington, New Zealand

Nachemson, A. (1991) Lumbar intradiscal pressure. In *The Lumbar Spine and Back Pain* (ed. M. I. V. Jayson), Pitman Medical, London

Pheasant, S. (1986) *Body Space. Anthropometry, Ergonomics and Design*, Taylor and Francis, London

Pheasant, S. (1991) *Ergonomics, Work and Health*, Taylor and Francis, London

Romiszowski, A. J. (1970) *Systems Approaches to Education and Training*, Kogan Page, London

Shackel, B. and Whitfield, D. (1969) General framework and workstation analysis. *Applied Ergonomics*, **1**, 33–41

Singleton, W. T. (1982) *The Body at Work*, Biological Ergonomics, Cambridge University Press, Cambridge

Spear, R. (1980) Systems approach to safety. *The World of Physical Risk*, Open University Press, Milton Keynes

van Wely, P. (1970) Design and disease. *Applied Ergonomics*, **1**, 262–269

Wilson, J. (1991) Participation – a framework and a foundation for ergonomics? *Journal of Occupational Psychology*, **64**, 67–80

Chapter 6

Occupational stress

Barbara Richardson

Introduction

There is wide-ranging literature which looks at mental stress and the individual. It is fascinating, complex and inconclusive – particularly with regard to occupational stress. Nevertheless, current theories of stress do help to throw light on some of the strategies which can be employed usefully in attempts to reduce or eliminate stress and, as such, warrant some scrutiny by physiotherapists in occupational health. Mental stress symptoms are 'less respectable' (Handy, 1993) than musculoskeletal stress ones but as all physiotherapists, who deal with the problems of musculoskeletal stress, are aware, mental stress can contribute greatly to the build-up and maintenance of musculoskeletal stress.

We spend long periods of our lives at work. '. . . it is a central activity of life, the basis of identity and a source of satisfaction and dissatisfaction' (Argyle, 1981). Well-being at work has been described as 'a dynamic state of mind characterized by reasonable harmony between a worker's ability, needs, expectations, environmental demands and opportunities' (Sutherland and Cooper, 1990). Each person will expect different rewards or benefits from work and have different abilities to cope with its demands. These may or may not match with the reality of work. As a consequence, work can influence well-being or mental stress levels. Management of musculoskeletal disorders and their consequences should have a broad base and look at the job–person fit from a physical as well as psychological point of view; in the clinical situation it is necessary to determine how much of the patient's symptoms are possibly related to mental stress.

Mental stress and its consequences

Mental stress is a difficult subject to study because it is not the components of the event but the individual's appraisal of it which is important. It is regarded variously as a stimulus, a response and as a perceived threat. The stimulus or challenge which spurs an individual to act to achieve a goal may be defined as a stress. An individual may be said to respond with stress to events in his or her surroundings. Events in an individual's surroundings such as a person, or a situation or challenge, which are perceived to be too demanding, may also be defined as stressful.

As is widely recorded (Cox, 1978; Cooper and Payne, 1991; Warr, 1991; Warren, 1992a), study of stress and individuals has taken differing approaches. The physiological model of stress proposed by Selye in the 1950s known as the *general adaptation syndrome* (Burns, 1991) identifies stages of the physiological stress response in body tissues engendered by the 'fight or flight' mechanism. An initial alarm reaction triggers the sympathetic response in preparation for action. If this does not take place and the situation persists, then the body attempts to resist the high catecholamine levels and their effects by adapting to them, and in doing so produces such symptoms as headaches, diarrhoea, muscle tension, sweating and sleeping problems, etc. Further persistence of the stress response eventually depletes the adaptive reserves of the tissues and full disease results.

The *psychological model of stress* proposed by Lazarus and others in the 1970s (Burns, 1991) contrasts with the physiological model of stress response and considers stress to be a stimulus. Stress is seen as a subjective experience which is dependent upon the perception and cognitive appraisal of events by the individual. Stress is perceived and interpreted as a demand on the individual. In this model, coping strategies are used following an initial alarm, if the benefits of successful coping are acknowledged to be more desirable than leaving the situation unaltered. If these are successful the alarm state will subside. If unsuccessful then depression and withdrawal will follow. Successful coping strategies are those which increase knowledge, awareness and understanding of events. Feedback is considered to be important at all levels. Unsuccessful coping strategies result in short-term stress behaviours such as ignoring the situation or using palliative drugs such as cigarettes, sleeping pills or alcohol. If not checked, these behaviours may lead to long-term stress-related illnesses such as dependence on drugs and alcohol and possibly cancer.

An *interactive model of stress* (Sutherland and Cooper, 1990) which draws together the underlying features of both physiological and psychological models and considers the stressor source, the perception of the situation and the response, is now put forward as the most useful in tackling stress. Mental stress can be stimulating or harmful. 'Being alive is synonymous with responding to stress' (Sutherland and Cooper, 1990) and it is that which provides the spur for healthy motivation, development and change. However, it can also be unmanageable, the cause of much misery and damaging to health. As Luoparjärvi (1985) pointed out, epidemiological investigations on health and well-being have defined the functional capacity of an individual as an entity of physical, mental and social capacities. Attempts to balance the demands of the working environment and different components of the individual's capabilities will go a long way towards protecting the individual from mental stress and promote well-being at work.

Mental stress of occupation

Warr (1991) distinguished context-free mental health from that which is job-related. Stress at work can result from many factors and combinations of factors. These include psychological factors concerned with job satisfaction, job-related anxiety, job-related depression, as well as physical factors related to levels of noise, heat, dust and physical workload. Balanced against this is the ability of the individual to relax after work. As Grandjean (1988) emphasized, the total stresses of mental and physical effort, problems and fatigue must be balanced by total recuperation within the 24-hour cycle. Much stress engendered in work can be diminished by leisure activities outside work. Equally, the stress of occupation can be compounded by further stress produced at home. This might be from internal family relationships, or activities in carrying out another job or taking other demanding roles in the community.

Factors which are accepted as influencing the mental stress level of people at work are time pressures, role ambiguity, role conflict, uncertainty at organizational boundaries, lack of job security, and poor relationships with the boss, colleagues or subordinates (Warr, 1991). Mental stress level is seen to be determined by the interaction between the person and the environment and to arise if environmental features are perceived as threatening. A threatening environment may be posed by the work activity itself, or the organization and conditions of the job.

With regard to the actual work activity, it is possible for the energy of heavy physical labour and the level of physiological stress in maintaining output to be assessed, however, new technology relies more on information processing and it is not so easy to assess 'cognitive' aspects of work, nor the individual's appraisal of it. Jobs which have a heavy cognitive load for the individual can lead to mental stress. Stress of this kind often first becomes noticeable in the deterioration of so-called secondary tasks – the inability to talk or to look out for hazards whilst undertaking the job. Increased error rate, accidents and fatigue can all be a sign of mental overload which may lead to mental stress. Similarly, pacing stress, where the individual may be acting at a rate faster or slower than his natural rhythm, may be very significant in types of work such as conveyor belt, group or piece-work, etc., or may even arise from demands placed on the individual which are external to work. Shift work, particularly night shifts, is another important potential source of mental stress. Each person has a natural circadian (biological) rhythm of approximately 25 hours in which heart rate and hormone secretion is regulated. There is a natural increase of adrenalin in the morning and a decrease at night (Folkard, 1991; McPherson 1993). Ideal shift lengths are of 8 hours or less, to give no time for the body to adjust the biological rhythms and to allow for continuity of family lifestyle to some extent. Ideal shift rotation intervals would be short-term with single, isolated night shifts each followed immediately by a full 24 hours' rest (Grandjean, 1988).

Organization and conditions of work are recognized as contributing to the overall satisfaction of doing a job. The two-factor theory of Herzberg (mid 1960s) is given much credence (see for example Handy, 1993; Warr, 1991). It proposes that job satisfaction is not the same as job dissatisfaction. Job satisfaction depends on factors that are specific to the individual such as the perceived freedom to choose, responsibility, levels of skill ability, variety of tasks, identification with the job, feedback on performance, being valued. Job dissatisfaction, however, is determined by factors such as pay, working conditions, hours of work, job security. In terms of sources of occupational stress, both aspects of work may be contributory, depending on the attitudes, aspirations and role of the individual.

Role problems can also produce individual tension, low morale or poor communication. *Role theory* (Handy, 1993; Sutherland and Cooper, 1990) looks at workers as members of an organization, groups and pairs. Roles signal the kind of contribution expected from each individual and the quality and quantity of the work required can produce a role stress, which can be a healthy role pressure or an unhealthy role strain. The individual may be overloaded with too many roles such as worker, health and safety officer and shop steward, or be underloaded with roles when having the capacity to be stretched further. There is a common myth that occupational stress is inherent in the managerial role but roles that have high demands and low autonomy, such as in unskilled or semi-skilled work, are also known to be stressful (Creed, 1993).

Roles may conflict within work, such as that of being both shop steward and supervisor, or the work role may seriously conflict with the home role. For example middle-aged women may be expected to maintain the full role of housekeeper, cook and cleaner in addition to the role demanded at work and may not receive the family support which is enjoyed by women from younger generations, who seem to share roles of home-making more readily (A. Eastlake, 1993, personal communication). Another source of role stress which can arise within the working group is a lack of role definition. A lack of congruence between the expectations of roles can lead to misinterpretations and much stress and frustration to the individual.

As reported by Renault de Moraes (1993), the *job characteristics questionnaire* of Hackman and Oldham and Cooper's *occupational stress indicator* are two attempts at trying to combine and quantify the overall occupational stress of an individual. Whilst the former looks more at factors external to the individual at work, the latter highlights the specific feelings of the individual about his or her job. Application of both may be a useful organizational strategy on occasions; however, on a day-to-day level, the physiotherapist in occupational health needs a good general overview of the behaviour and abilities of people in response to stress and the problems of daily life in order to plan appropriate intervention.

Individuals and occupational stress

An undertanding of the variety of ways individuals perceive and cope with potential stress of work and the working environment is central to effective management of stress. Cooper and Payne (1991) went to great lengths to emphasize the role of individual differences in stress perception and response. Creed (1993) believes that there has been inadequate research relating personality and other variables to stress at work. However, it is generally accepted that personality characteristics, traits and disposition play an important part in the relationship between job demands and worker health. Current research (Sutherland and Cooper 1990; Cooper and Payne, 1991; Laungani, 1993) looks at parameters of self esteem, introversion/extroversion and rigid and flexible personalities in relation to coping with stress. Theory of *type A behaviour patterns* (TABP), first identified by Friedman and Rosenman in the mid 1970s in relation to coronary heart disease, and the *locus of control* (LOC) theory of Rotter (mid 1960s) are receiving most attention.

TABP theory has a firm link with coronary heart disease, although it is still being challenged (Sutherland and Cooper, 1990). 'Type A' people may be found in all walks of life; the majority are male but type A has also been found in the female population and even type A nuns have been identified. The person who exhibits a type A behaviour is considered to be more prone to stress. Behavioural elements include an exaggerated sense of time, excessive competitiveness and striving for achievement, hostility and aggressiveness. These types of behaviours may be compounded by a situation at work and the concept is used in considering employee–job fit and the self-selected occupations of individuals. In a work setting, such people will constantly work long hours to reach deadlines in conditions of work overload, will take work home and will feel misunderstood and show exasperation to work colleagues. In response to demand they will always pace faster to get more done and will have difficulty in relaxing and winding down.

The degree of control individuals think they have over what happens to them is thought to be a very important factor in the mitigation of stressful situations (Hurrell and Murphy, 1991). LOC theory proposes that people vary in whether they believe the outcomes of life are due to their own internal personal abilities or caused by factors outside their control such as fate, chance, and other people. Those who see themselves having control over their environment (an internal locus of control) display more hardiness and are less likely to show anxiety under stress than those who feel they have little control over their environment (external locus of control). For example, if new equipment or technology is introduced at work it is likely that 'externals' will be more reluctant to change and to use it then the 'internals' who will be curious to explore it (Sutherland and Cooper, 1990).

Other mediating factors in responding to stress are information or prior experience of events, which allows a prediction of one's own behaviour and how one will be affected, and social support. Social support plays a key role. Support may be recognized as feedback or emotional. The Holmes and Rahe *social re-adjustment rating scale* for predicting stress levels ranks and compounds the significance of life's events (see O'Neill, 1988). It may be a helpful indicator of the potential for stress, although it is controversial as people react to life's situations according to the meanings they have for them individually. The social climate of a working group can offer a strong support and solace to modify the effects of occupational stress for the individual.

Physiotherapy intervention

Intervention is aimed at changing the job or helping the individual to cope. As suggested by Warr (1991), stress management may require arrangements which give the worker more opportunity for control over his affairs, for skill use and to be involved with the organization of the job. It may require giving more understanding of the overall job design. Issues such as physical security, or availability of money, or a lack of opportunity for interpersonal contact, or a feeling of being in an undervalued social position may lie at the roots of the stress. In some situations, and with a sympathetic management, job redesign, job enrichment or job reorganization may be possible. If this is not the case, the particular characteristics of the individual will determine the coping strategies which should be adopted and their likely level of success.

It is necessary to consider if the coping mechanisms already in use are helping or hindering the individual. Cooperative solutions and establishing 'stability zones' (Handy, 1993) which include proper rest, recreation and outside stimulus are of most value. Rationalization and accepting conflicts as inevitable and to be lived with, are also healthy coping mechanisms to be encouraged. However, coping strategies may result in unilateral solutions such as taking the stress into the home and creating problems for others elsewhere, or withdrawal, which may take the form of avoidance or containing the stress within the self, with physiological consequences.

It is these psychophysiological pathways of stress response that form the basis of many of the problems encountered in a physiotherapy department (Warren, 1992a) in occupational health. They may present either in the form of musculoskeletal symptoms or in association with them. People may or may not be aware of the contribution of occupational stress to their symptoms or of how they are coping with it. Pain is subject to modification not only by the conditioned threshold to pain of the individual, established through the processes of cultural and familial socialization, but also by factors which will lower it or raise it on a day-to-day basis. These include the conscious or unconscious awareness of the significance of role: 'getting the job done'; motivation; ambitions; need for drawing attention to the self; and need for the use of pain in drawing attention to or away from other anxieties perceived by the individual (Bond, 1984; French, 1992). Very often, attending for treatment itself may be stressful since it implies that the worker may not be working at full strength. People may have unreasonable anxieties about losing their jobs or about losing money if they are not able to attend work. It must also be remembered that some ethnic groups and the lower socio-economic groups, especially those with a poor education, tend to present emotional difficulties in the form of physical symptoms (Scambler, 1992). Whilst in the 'sick role' (Scambler, 1991), the individual is freed from the usual responsibilities of life at home and at work, and sometimes this may be welcomed as a protection against the stresses produced by the responsibilities of everyday life or conflicts at work.

Many people feel they are trapped in their predicament and that there are no alternative means of perceiving their situation. They feel there are no choices. Readjustment of a person's view and an insight into difficulties may often be facilitated by the occupational health physiotherapist during the treatment interaction (Saunders and Maxwell, 1988). A better perspective on the problem can be gained through a clearer definition of priorities and purposes. The physiotherapist can help by establishing a helping relationship in which thoughts and feelings can be expressed in such a way as to come to terms with a new situation or see troubling situations more objectively. This sort of 'indirect counselling' (Egan, 1975) as a professional activity is a process which moves markedly away from directing others and much more to encouraging the individual to direct him/herself. The relationship is empathetic, respectful and genuine and includes paying attention to non-verbal communication, listening skills, probing, reflection and finally helping the individual to find the theme of the disclosures through the use of paraphrasing and summarizing (Thomson, 1992).

Utilizing mediating factors known to help coping strategies such as information and social support is important in stress management. Relaxation techniques, particularly those which can be used in the work situation, can also be of use in reinforcing coping mechanisms and offer some measure of self-control for the individual. Roskies (1991) proposed the use of physical exercise as a stress buffer although she pointed out that, paradoxically, exercise as a mental health strategy is often the choice for individuals not already overburdened by stress and it is those who are who may resort to smoking or alcohol as a stress buffer. It may also be appropriate on occasions to take a behaviour modification approach against abnormal illness behaviour, as recommended by Williams (1989) and Warren (1992b).

Intervention in the workplace rather than within the individual may be more problematic but it should be possible to solve conflicts between the mental health needs of employees and the productivity requirements of management with or without the help of industrial relations. Often only minor changes in work need be made. Rest breaks which would help to mitigate pacing stress, for example, need not be long and often a change of activity or scene is all that is required. Ten-minute breaks may be ample if taken regularly, allowing interaction with others socially or to give a change of view.

Management should be encouraged to recognize the special problems of working with new technology in a proactive manner. Guidelines for the introduction of visual display technology (Kalimo and Leppänen, 1987) could usefully have a more general application for the introduction of any new technology. These recognize the problems of introducing a technology which is entirely new and unknown for many, particularly the older age group, and acknowledge a resistance to organizational change and the fear of being de-skilled and less qualified in the eyes of work colleagues or, conversely, the frustrations of being over-qualified for work which has become more monotonous and isolating. As well as giving attention to posture to reduce stress on eyes, neck and back, etc., the physiotherapist could profitably encourage the new work to be of an adjustable pace; an even workload which does not depend on others, and which gives opportunity to influence its organization and to spend time with others. It is also important to ensure that the employee has knowledge of the whole work process and the functioning of the equipment.

With the continual introduction of new technologies and the changes in jobs entailed, occupational stress is likely to become a more rather than less prominent feature of working life in the future. It does impinge on the work of the physiotherapist in occupational health both by its direct association with physiological responses of the individual, which may create disorders or may impede progress in the treatment of other conditions, and by its more indirect effects on the general health and well-being of groups of workers. A practical knowledge of changing work processes and work demands in an organization, combined with sensitive appreciation of workers' individual needs and responses and good communication with management, can give the physiotherapist a powerful tool with which to combat occupational stress to the benefit of the individual worker and the organization as a whole.

Occupational stress 81

References

Argyle, M. (1981) *The Social Psychology of Work*, Pelican, Middlesex

Bond, M. R. (1984) *Pain, Its Nature, Analysis and Treatment*, Churchill Livingstone, Edinburgh

Burns, R. B. (1991) *Essential Psychology*, MTP Press, Lancaster

Cooper, C. L. and Payne, R. (1991) *Personality and Stress: Individual Differences in the Stress Process*, John Wiley, Chichester

Cox, T. (1978) *Stress*, Macmillan Press, London

Creed, F. (1993) Mental health problems at work. *Student British Medical Journal*, **1**, 317–318

Egan, G. (1975) *The Skilled Helper*, Brooks/Cole, Monterey, California

Folkard, S. (1991) Circadian rhythms and hours of work. In *Psychology at Work*, 4th edn (ed. P. Warr), Pelican, Middlesex

French, S. (1992) The psychology and sociology of pain. In *Physiotherapy: A Psychosocial Approach* (ed. S. French), Butterworth–Heinemann, Oxford

Grandjean, E. (1988) *Fitting the Task to the Man*. Taylor and Francis, London

Handy, C. B. (1993) *Understanding Organisations*, Penguin, Middlesex

Hurrell, J. J. and Murphy, L. R. (1991) Locus of control, job demands and health. In *Personality and Stress: Individual Differences in the Stress Process*. John Wiley, Chichester

Kalimo, R. and Leppänen, A. (1987) Visual display units – psychosocial factors in health. In *Women and Technology* (ed. M. T. Davidson and C. L. Cooper), John Wiley, Chichester

Laungani, P. (1993) Cultural differences in stress and its management. *Stress Medicine*, **9**, 37–43

Luoparjärvi, T. (1985) Interaction of workload and functional capacity. In *Ergonomics International '85* (eds I. D. Brown, R. Goldsmith, K. Coombes and M. A. Sinclair), proceedings of 9th Congress of International Ergonomic Association (Bournemouth, 1985), Taylor and Francis, London

McPherson, G. (1993) Shiftwork and the offshore worker. *Occupational Health*, **45**, 237–239

O'Neill, E. (1988) Change is the key to stress. *Physiotherapy*, **74**, 429–434

Renault de Moraes, (1993) A study of occupational stress among government white-collar workers in Brazil using the occupational stress indicator. *Stress Medicine* **9**, 91–104

Roskies, E. (1991) Individual differences in health behaviour. In

Personality and Stress: Individual Differences in the Stress Process (ed. C. L. Cooper and R. Payne), J Wiley, Chichester

Saunders, C. and Maxwell, M. (1988) The case for counselling in physiotherapy. *Physiotherapy*, **74**, 592–596

Scambler, A. (1992) Ethnicity, health and health care. In *Physiotherapy: A Psychosocial Approach* (ed. S. French), Butterworth–Heinemann, Oxford

Scambler, G. (1991) Health and illness behaviour. In *Sociology as Applied to Medicine* (ed. G. Scambler), Baillière Tindall, London

Sutherland, V. and Cooper, C. L. (1990) *Understanding Stress*, Chapman and Hall, London

Thomson, D. (1992) Counselling. In *Physiotherapy: A Psychosocial Approach* (ed. S. French), Butterworth–Heinemann, Oxford

Warr, P. (1991) Job characteristics and mental health. In *Psychology at Work*, 4th edn (ed. P. Warr), Pelican, Middlesex

Warren, E. (1992a) Psychophysiological and somatoform disorders. In *Physiotherapy: A Psychosocial Approach* (ed. S. French), Butterworth–Heinemann, Oxford

Warren, E. (1992b) Psychological treatment in physiotherapy practice. In *Physiotherapy: A Psychosocial Approach* (ed. S. French), Butterworth–Heinemann, Oxford

Williams, J. (1989) Illness to wellness behaviour. *Physiotherapy*, **75**, 2–7

Further reading

Fletcher, B. C. (1991) *Work, Stress, Disease and Life Expectancy*, John Wiley, Chichester

Chapter 7

Anatomy and physiology of movement at work

Nancy M. Laurenson

Introduction

Physical movement, especially in the working environment, has changed dramatically in the past two centuries. In Western society and culture today there is less emphasis and need placed upon motor skills and physical exertion in the working conditions which present to most people. This is in sharp contrast to the daily routine of heavy manual labour still found in developing countries.

Exercise is considered to be of benefit to people (Royal College of Physicians of London, 1991; Fentem et al., 1992; Sports Council and Health Education Authority, 1992), yet it may be questioned if this benefit applies to those in some manual working conditions in achieving a certain quality of life. As the tradition of physical or manual work shifts to a more technological and thus sedentary way of life, physical exercise tends to be encountered only in leisure activities and sport. Many individuals work to get fit rather than become fit to do work or enjoy leisure activities. This dilemma can pose many problems, not least cycles of injury and re-injury as well as safety issues. In the workplace it is important to recognize the variations between individuals in their ability to perform and adapt to different modes of work and to consider how this may be enhanced or constrained by lifestyles adopted away from the workplace.

Bioenergetics

The ability to perform work depends on many factors but ultimately this is achieved by the ability of the muscle cell to transform chemical energy in the form of food (fuel) into mechanical energy for muscular work utilizing energy-yielding processes in the muscle cell. Movement occurs because of activation (contraction) of skeletal muscle which accounts for 25–35% of body weight in the average adult woman and 40–45% in the average adult man. The immediate energy source for all metabolic processes including muscle activation is adenosine triphosphate (ATP). In addition, movement and physical work require large quantities of fuel and oxygen for the transformation and release of energy in skeletal muscles. The extent and scale of the change in rate of transformation during heavy physical work or exercise may rise from a resting metabolic rate of approximately 1 kcal.min^{-1} (4.2 kJ) in a 70 kg person to 20 kcal.min^{-1} or more during heavy exertion. Table 7.1 outlines a classification system which is based on the energy requirements of untrained men and women performing different tasks. Daily energy expenditure based on dietary surveys of nutrient intake for various occupational groups of different ages is shown in Table 7.2. It is wise to point out the wide variability in rates. This is largely explained by the intensity and duration of activities performed outside work, especially those related to leisure pursuits or physical exercise.

The physiological challenge of exertion involves not only the provision of fuel and oxygen to maintain rates of energy transformation, but the ability to remove the waste products of metabolism and carbon dioxide and heat. The chemical reactions which take place within each cell and allow for energy transfer are well described in McArdle et al. (1991) and Åstrand and Rodahl (1986), and are summarized in Fig. 7.1. The adenosine triphosphate – adenosine diphosphate (ATP–ADP) system represents the fundamental carrier of chemical energy in every cellular reaction. The major energy pathway for ATP production and breakdown differs depending on the type of fuel present as well as the intensity and duration of the work. In intense exercise of short duration (lifting loads,

Table 7.1 Classification of physical activity in terms of exercise intensity

	Energy expenditure							
	Men				Women			
Level	kcal.min^{-1}	l.min^{-1}	ml.kg^{-1}.min^{-1}	MET	kcal.min^{-1}	l.min^{-1}	ml.kg^{-1}.min^{-1}	MET
Light	2.0–4.9	0.40–0.99	6.1–15.2	1.6–3.9	1.5–3.4	0.30–0.69	5.4–12.5	1.2–2.7
Moderate	5.0–7.4	1.00–1.49	15.3–22.9	4.0–5.9	3.5–5.4	0.70–1.09	12.6–19.8	2.8–4.3
Heavy	7.5–9.9	1.50–1.99	23.0–30.6	6.0–7.9	5.5–7.4	1.10–1.49	19.9–27.1	4.4–5.9
Very heavy	10.0–12.4	2.00–2.49	30.7–38.3	8.0–9.9	7.5–9.4	1.50–1.89	27.2–34.4	6.0–7.5
Unduly heavy	12.5–	2.50–	38.4–	10.0–	9.5–	1.90–	34.5–	7.6–

l.min^{-1} based on 5 kcal per litre of oxygen; ml.kg^{-1}.min^{-1} based on a 65 kg man and a 55 kg woman; one MET (metabolic equivalent of the task) is equivalent to the average resting oxygen consumption from McArdle et al. (1991).

Table 7.2 Daily rates of energy expenditure for various occupations kcal.day^{-1}

	Energy expenditure (kcal.day^{-1})		
Occupation	Average	Minimum	Maximum
Men			
Elderly retired	2330	1750	2810
Office workers	2520	1820	3270
Coal mine clerks	2800	2330	3290
Laboratory technicians	2840	2240	3820
Older industrial workers	2840	2180	3710
University students	2930	2270	4410
Building workers	3000	2440	3730
Steel workers	3280	2600	3960
Army cadets	3490	2990	4100
Older peasants (Swiss)	3530	2210	5000
Farmers	3550	2450	4670
Coal miners	3660	2970	4560
Forestry workers	3670	2860	4600
Women			
Older housewives	1990	1490	2410
Middle-aged housewives	2090	1760	2320
Laboratory assistants	2130	1340	2540
Assistants in department store	2250	1820	2850
University students	2290	2090	2500
Factory workers	2320	1970	2980
Bakery workers	2510	1980	3390
Older peasants (Swiss)	2890	2200	3860

From Durnin and Passmore (1967).

sprinting) the energy is derived from stored intramuscular ATP and creatine phosphate. As intense exercise continues the energy is produced primarily from anaerobic glycolysis. This short-term energy system is limited due to the increasing lactate levels which are a byproduct of anaerobic glycolysis. When lactate rises above a tolerable level it can inhibit muscle contraction. This level varies for each individual depending on their training status. In comparison, in endurance activities of long duration such as hill walking or, for example,

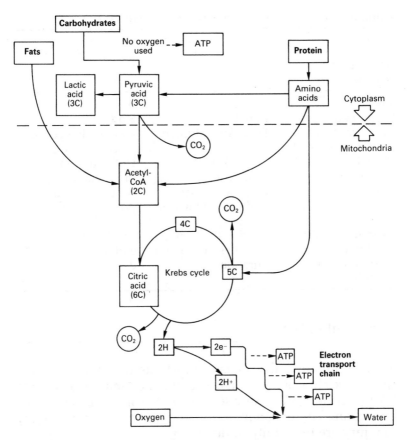

Fig. 7.1 Organic compounds containing carbon and hydrogen (fats, carbohydrates, proteins) may be totally combusted to carbon dioxide (CO_2) and water by oxygen, that is, by the process of a catalytic oxidation with the aid of enzymes in the living cell. For some of the steps the numbers of carbon atoms involved are given. ADP, adenosine diphosphate; ATP, adenosine triphosphate. From Åstrand and Rodahl (1986).

loading and unloading tasks, aerobic metabolism predominates and makes use of oxygen which is available to the cell; energy is then produced in the mitochondria utilizing glycogen, glucose or free fatty acids as a fuel source. Energy exchange in muscles is summarized in Table 7.3.

Table 7.3 General characteristics of the energy systems

	System	
ATP–creatine phosphate	*Lactic acid*	*Oxygen*
Anaerobic	Anaerobic	Aerobic
Very rapid	Rapid	Slow
Chemical fuel: creatine phosphate	Food fuel: glycogen	Food fuel: glycogen, glucose, fats, protein
Very limited ATP production	Limited ATP production	Unlimited ATP production
Muscular stores limited	By-product lactic acid causes muscular fatigue	No fatiguing by-products
Used with sprint or any high-powered, short duration activities	Used with intense activities of 1–3 min duration	Used with endurance or long duration activities

Muscle fibre types

Skeletal muscle is the focus of most attention when discussing work physiology. Thus, knowing how muscle responds to the challenge of exercise is essential if the mechanisms underlying fatigue, adaptations to training and vulnerability to injury are to be fully understood.

Skeletal muscle fibres exist in a state of passive (resting) or active (contracting) form. It is the activation of muscle as the essential event which allows for movement and thus work to be performed. However, the decision to move a particular muscle is only accomplished in a complex, yet very specific sequence of electrical and chemical reactions which result in the mechanical displacement of the actin and myosin protein myofilaments lying within the muscle sarcomere. The sliding filament theory of muscle contraction as proposed by A.F. Huxley (1974) is now widely accepted. The myosin strands that comprise a body and head (see Fig. 7.2) point towards the actin proteins. The tropomyosin molecule, linked to the actin strand, is found where the myosin interacts with the

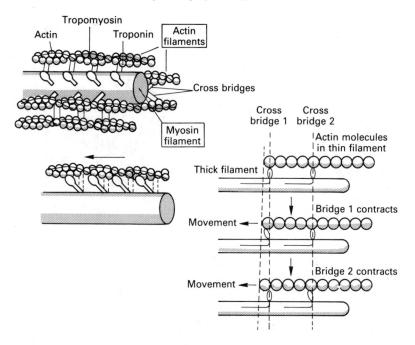

Fig. 7.2 Relative positioning of actin and myosin filaments during the oscillating movement of the cross bridges. The action of each bridge contributes a small displacement of movement. For clarity, one of the actin strands is omitted from the left-hand figure. The myosin ATPase is located on the globular heads of the myosin; this 'active' head frees the energy from ATP to be used in muscle contraction. From McArdle et al. (1991).

actin. This molecule acts as a blocking agent between the natural affinity of actin and myosin. When calcium is released from the sarcoplasmic reticulum, in response to a nerve impulse, it binds to troponin and a complex twisting movement occurs which extricates the tropomyosin molecule and allows the myosin head to attach itself to actin. Almost immediately, energy is released by ATP breakdown.

Two primary types of motor units have been identified and classified by their contractile and metabolic characteristics. These are slow-fatiguing Type I fibres and fast-fatiguing Types IIa and IIb fibres. Figure 7.3 demonstrates the differences between the fibre types, highlighting not only fibre size, twitch response and fatigue curves, but the metabolic

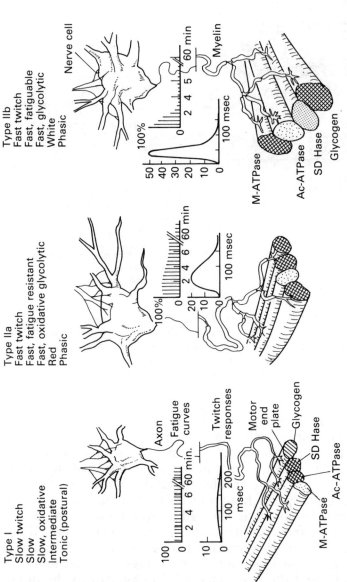

Fig. 7.3 In adult mammalian muscles, microscopic examination after transverse (cross) sectioning and histological staining reveals three fibre types. Fibres are classified as either type I (slow) or type II (fast), depending on intensity of staining with alkaline myofibrillar (M) ATPase. Note that type I and II fibres demonstrate an 'acid reverse' when stained for myofibrillar ATPase at low pH (Ac-ATPase). With the oxidative marker succinic dehydrogenase (SDH), type I and type IIa fibres stain dark, whereas type IIb fibres stain lightly. Glycogen content is revealed by the periodic acid Schiff (PAS) stain. The three fibre types differ in ease of recruitment, metabolism, twitch characteristics and rate of fatigue. The alternative terminologies used to classify skeletal muscle fibre types are indicated at the top. From Edington and Edgerton (1976).

Type I
Slow twitch
Slow
Slow, oxidative
Intermediate
Tonic (postural)

Type IIa
Fast twitch
Fast, fatigue resistant
Fast, oxidative glycolytic
Red
Phasic

Type IIb
Fast twitch
Fast, fatiguable
Fast, glycolytic
White
Phasic

Nerve cell

Myelin

Axon

Fatigue curves

Twitch responses

Motor end plate

Glycogen

SD Hase

Ac-ATPase

M-ATPase

Ac-ATPase

SD Hase

Glycogen

M-ATPase

differences when examining histochemical stains for appropriate enzymes. Prolonged low intensity exercise or postural use of muscles is supported almost entirely by Type I fibres with some use of Type IIa. As exercise intensity increases during activities such as lifting or pushing heavy weights or running at fast speeds, Type II fibres are brought more and more into use. During maximal exercise all fibres are recruited. This recruitment takes place in a hierarchical manner whereby Type I fibres are always recruited first followed by Type IIa and then IIb fibres as the tension reaches a maximum.

Type I muscles fibres are designed to make maximum use of aerobic metabolism to support their prolonged periods of activity. These fibres have a good capillary supply; their mitochondria provide the cellular framework for the aerobic conversion of energy from carbohydrate and fatty acid breakdown into ATP. It is not surprising then, that the aerobic capacity of a muscle is improved by a training-induced increase in capillary and mitochondrial density, as seen in any endurance activity such as swimming and cycling or low-weight, high-repetition weight training. Type II fibres rely on the anaerobic pathway for energy provision and suffer the consequences of lactic acid accumulation. In a work environment where static exercise using small muscle groups is employed the build-up of lactic acid is minor and does not appear to be a limiting factor in total work rate. However, the decrease in blood flow and the accumulation of metabolites may cause a localized muscle pain. The mitochondrial density of the Type II fibres is low; however, the Type IIa fibres will respond to endurance training by increasing their complement of mitochondria and become less fatiguable. In this sense these 'intermediate' fibres are more closely related to Type I fibres in their metabolic potential.

Characteristics of muscle action

The maximal tension that any muscle fibre can develop is influenced by several factors. The force produced is dependent on the relative length of the muscle fibre at the time of the

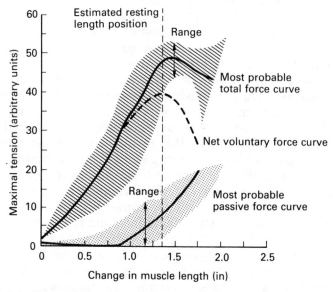

Fig. 7.4 Isometric force-length data for human triceps muscle. To obtain the net voluntary force curve the values from the passive force curve were subtracted from the total force curve. From Åstrand and Rodahl (1986).

contraction. The tension reaches a maximum at a relative length of about 1.2:1 and decreases at lower and higher lengths. Figure 7.4 depicts a length–tension curve for a human muscle. It shows clearly that in a work situation there is an optimal length at which the muscle fibre responds when force is exerted against an external resistance. The contractile components of skeletal muscle can increase by an amazing 67% from their resting length (Alter, 1988). This enables the muscle to move through a wide range of motion. Functional movement develops due to the collaboration of different muscles acting in a synergistic fashion as the limb changes position. Thus, movement occurs, as the lever arms in the body through which the muscle forces are transformed into pulls and pushes, alter with the changing positions of movable joints.

Figure 7.5 illustrates the classic force–velocity curve. This well-known S-shaped relationship highlights the variation in

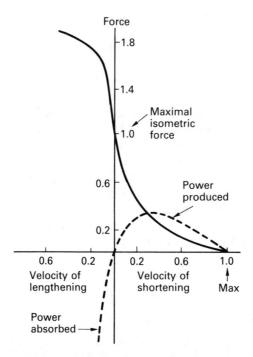

Fig. 7.5 Classical force–velocity curve (full line) obtained on an isolated muscle, showing the maximal force that can be developed when a muscle is contracting at various speeds. Note that the maximal force in a concentric activity is less than in an isometric contraction. Highest force can be attained in a rapid eccentric contraction. The dotted line gives the maximal power, i.e. the force times the velocity of contraction. Curves differ according to the muscles studied. In in vivo experiments, the analysis is complicated because in movements, the muscles are rarely contracting isotonically; the leverage changes during a dynamic contraction and therefore the force demand on a muscle is not constant even when the external load is kept constant. From Åstrand and Rodahl (1986).

maximal force developed by muscles during contraction at different speeds. The highest force which can be developed occurs in a fast eccentric contraction; this force declines to a minimum when the muscle is activated at high speeds in a concentric contraction. Thus, speed of contraction is important to control when determining dynamic strength. Electromyographic studies have shown that the degree of muscle excitation required to produce a given force of contraction is smaller when the active muscle is forcibly stretched than when the muscle shortens at the same velocity. Studies (Åstrand and Rodahl, 1986) have also shown that during work at comparative rates, oxygen demand (oxygen uptake) is much less during eccentric compared with concentric contractions.

The force of muscle contraction can thus be stated to be dependent on several factors: (1) number and size of motor unit firing; (2) rate of firing of individul motor units; (3) composition of motor units; (4) velocity of muscle shortening; (5) length of muscle fibre; (6) condition of muscle fibre; and (7) age of muscle fibre. Therefore, good motivation, skill, position, speed of movement, muscle condition and muscle age should all be of concern for an optimal work activity and in planning training programmes.

Training

Training for physical activity of any type should be based on principles of adaptation and progressive overload. As a general rule, it is important to keep in mind the specific purpose of the training; the best training is achieved simply by carrying out the activity itself. The goals following training or conditioning should be to reduce energy demands at submaximal work loads and to increase total energy output capability at maximum exercise.

Physical training should expose the individual to a work stress that can be defined in terms of intensity, frequency and duration to produce a measurable training effect or improvement in function. In order for further improvement to take place, the training intensity must be increased, producing an overload effect. Thus, the more fit a person is the more it will take to improve upon that fitness. Unfortunately, the exact magnitude of the training load necessary to produce an optimal effect is not established (Åstrand and Rodahl, 1986), but will vary between individuals and be dependent on factors such as age and current training status or fitness. Improvements are found to be greatest in sedentary individuals.

Training for muscle strength produces adaptations to

skeletal muscle which can be classified as either neurogenic, i.e. those changes which occur in the motor neuron, or myogenic, i.e. those changes which occur in the muscle fibre structure. The neurogenic changes tend to be the first response: as a result of a specific resistance training programme a greater number of muscle fibres are recruited earlier and in a more synchronous manner. There is better overall organization and patterning of the motor unit, i.e. there is a learned response which involves better skill or technique in performing the movement. The myogenic changes, on the other hand, occur over time and are represented by actual changes in the muscle structure and metabolism. The cross-sectional area enlarges with the addition of sarcomeres, resulting in muscle hypertrophy. The mitochondria also tend to increase, as well as the number and variety of enzymes which help speed conversion of ATP or utilize energy or the fuel source more quickly.

In a weight-training programme or work situation which demands increased use of the arm muscles, for instance, the initial ability to lift heavier loads is due to neurogenic changes. The actual strength of the muscle has not increased, only the skill or technique involved in executing the movement. However, with continued training the muscle fibres would hypertrophy, increasing total cross-sectional area and producing myogenic changes. Muscle disuse which occurs due to injury, immobilization or bedrest, as well as ageing and general non-use will result in muscle atrophy and a reduced cross-sectional area of both Type I and II fibres. This atrophy can occur within a short time and in extreme cases may result in dramatic muscle tissue loss.

Work

Work can be defined in terms of energy expenditure (kcal min^{-1}) or oxygen consumption (l min^{-1}) as already noted in Table 7.1. It can also be expressed in units as follows:

1. Work (joules) $\equiv$ force $\times$ distance
   1 joule $\equiv$ 1 newton metre

2. Force (newtons) $\equiv$ mass $\times$ acceleration
   1 newton $\equiv$ 1 kg.metre^{-1}.s^{-2}
3. Power (watts) $\equiv$ work per unit of time, or the rate of performing work, i.e. force $\times$ velocity
   1 watt $\equiv$ 1 joule.s^{-1}.

However, work is best described by the action of muscles, i.e. static versus dynamic work. In static work a muscle produces a force although there is no change in length of the sarcomere. This action is often termed isometric and is seen in activities where a load is supported or braced or movement is prevented. A classic sporting description would be a tug-of-war between two teams of equal strength or an arm wrestling contest of the same description. Comparable industrial situations are to be found in many moving and handling activities or in the sustained pressures required of drilling, fitting or use of control manoeuvres. Since there is no movement or the distance is zero in an isometric contraction no mechanical work is done according to physical laws, yet isometric activity demands energy and can be very fatiguing. Dynamic work, on the other hand, involves repetitive muscle activation using both alternate eccentric and concentric or agonist/antagonist contractions, as seen in walking or arm swinging. Much of movement involves combinations of both dynamic and static work. A useful example is the description of an individual carrying a load while walking. A more extreme sporting form of this description would be a figure skater supporting a partner in a hold or lift while continuing skating.

Work can be assessed or measured in a variety of ways; however, testing of exercise or work capacity must be specific to the muscles which are used or the activity which is done. It is wise to remember that the results of different tests may not necessarily be well correlated. Generally, testing procedures which look at whole body demands of muscle groups involved in dynamic progressive exercise of rhythmic contractions are useful in measuring overall 'potential'. The muscle bulk involved in such tests must be large, i.e. running, walking uphill or cycling, in order to effect a cardiorespiratory response. If a small muscle group such as the arms only is involved, then it will generate a local physiological response which is different from that seen when testing a large muscle group, i.e. there will be an increased heart rate for any given amount of measured work.

Cardiovascular responses

Interest in the cardiovascular response to exercise is directed towards the mechanisms by which the system attempts to cope with the increased demands for oxygen transport to skeletal muscles and transport of waste products of metabolism, as well as the transport of heat to the periphery of the body for temperature regulation. The cardiovascular response to exercise (see Figure 7.6) involves an increase in

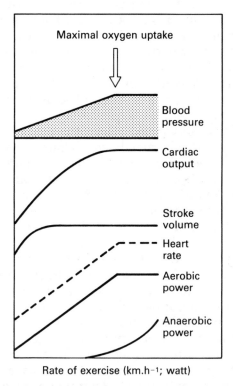

Fig. 7.6 Schematic diagram showing some of the major cardiovascular responses to exercise of increasing intensity. From Åstrand and Rodahl (1986).

cardiac output (the product of stroke volume and heart rate) and its redistribution to exercising skeletal muscle and to the skin. The redistribution of cardiac output to the working muscle occurs at the expense of the splanchnic and renal blood flow and can increase from approximately 15% of minute blood flow at rest to approximately 90% during maximum exercise.

As the workload becomes more demanding there is a linear increase in heart rate and oxygen consumption ($\dot{V}O_2$). As exercise progresses an individual will reach an intensity at which there is no further increase in oxygen consumption; this plateau is called the maximum oxygen uptake ($\dot{V}O_2$ max) and it is one of the important indicators of an individual's capability for sustained exercise or aerobic power. The $\dot{V}O_2$ max of an individual is genetically predetermined; however, with proper endurance training this value can be improved by up to 30% in formerly sedentary individuals.

The extent of cardiac output redistribution as well as any given measure of work can be determined by the relative exercise intensity. This is best described as the oxygen cost of an activity expressed as a percentage of an individual's maximum $\dot{V}O_2$ (%$\dot{V}O_2$max). Thus, the cardiovascular, thermoregulatory and even metabolic responses to work occur in proportion to the relative rather than absolute exercise intensity. This concept can be explained: if a random group of people are asked to run a mile in 8 min or unload a truck of beer barrels in a set amount of time, the absolute workload is the same for this group but the relative cost to each individual will vary. For some this may be an easy task and constitute a relative exercise intensity of possibly 60% $\dot{V}O_2$max. For others, the task may be extremely difficult and require a person to work at 85% of their $\dot{V}O_2$max. For still others, they may not be able to complete the task in the allotted time. It is most important to bear this concept in mind when prescribing training or work programmes or when making comparative measures between individuals.

Heart rate monitoring can be useful as a measure of exercise intensity and can be determined by palpating the radial or carotid artery pulse. For any given amount of physical activity, heart rate will lower as adaptation to work

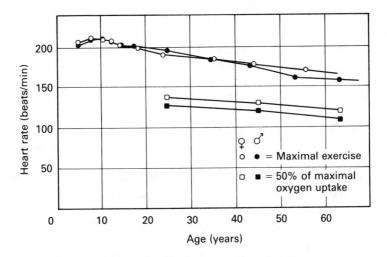

Fig. 7.7 Decline in maximal heart rate with age, and heart rate during a submaximal work rate; mean values from studies on 350 subjects. The standard deviation in maximal heart rate is about ±10 beats/min in all age groups. From Åstrand and Rodahl (1986).

occurs. This is also seen clearly when determining early morning or true resting pulse, which will lower as the heart becomes stronger. To maintain cardiac output, stroke volume must increase to compensate for the decrease in heart rate. Maximal heart rate declines with age and must be taken into account when determining accepted training or 'target' heart rates (Figure 7.7). It has been shown by the use of the Borg scale that subjective feelings of effort, commonly termed 'rate of perceived exertion', correlate well with heart rate and may be used as a general guide in determining individual effort (Åstrand and Rodahl, 1986i).

Fatigue

The mechanisms underlying fatigue during physical work are unclear and unlikely to be the result of one single limiting factor. Jones and Round (1990) have described the problems encountered when discussing the different meanings of fatigue. The sensations of tired, exhausted, overused, or the inability to 'go on' may occur due to a consequence of powerful muscular activity of a prolonged nature or one brief intensity coupled with powerful psychological and mental influences which cannot be overlooked. The multifactorial causes can be classified into peripheral or central factors which themselves are crucially dependent on the nature of the physical demands.

Peripheral fatigue can be identified according to changes that occur in the muscle due to large fluxes in metabolic concentration. These altered metabolic levels tend to affect muscle force production by actin and myosin and can be described as 'failure to maintain the required expected output' (Åstrand and Rodahl, 1986) or the inability to generate a specific force. Central fatigue can be defined as those mechanisms which occur at any of the links in the chain from the central command originating in the cortical or cerebellar brain centres to the sliding of actin and myosin filaments. Ultimately, fatigue can be defined as an energy crisis in the muscle cell where ATP hydrolysis does not equal ATP synthesis.

During high intensity or maximal exercise, fatigue in the muscle has been associated with insufficient ATP replenishment or the inhibition of ATP regeneration as a result of less calcium being available. It is also associated with a lowering of muscle pH due to hydrogen ion (H^+) accumulation in the sarcoplasm of the muscle cells as a result of anaerobic glycolysis. In addition, the accumulation of inorganic phosphate in the fatigued muscle might be expected to affect cross bridge cycling. There also appears to be a slowing of relaxation from an isometric contraction of acutely fatigued muscle. This slowing leads to a reduction in tetanic fusion frequency with a shift to the left of the force–frequency relationship (Figure 7.8). Evidence is gathering (Jones and Round, 1990) that a slowing of tetanic fusion frequency may be caused by two processes: 'decreased pH due to H^+ accumulation probably slows the cross bridge cycle while changes in phosphorus metabolites lead to a slow reaccumulation of calcium by the sarcoplasmic reticulum'. Finally, it has been suggested that increased potassium ion concentration in the

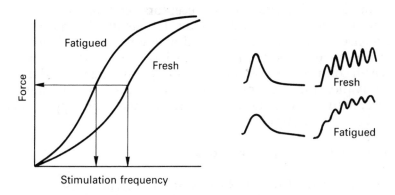

Fig. 7.8 Effect of slow relaxation in fatigued muscle on the force–frequency relationship. The insert shows the effect of fatigue on the degree of fusion; on the left, single twitches; on the right, stimulation at 7Hz. From Jones and Round (1990).

extracellular fluid may cause rapid force losses which slow the action potential conduction velocity. Research of this nature is important, as much of work involves isometric contractions in which local fatigue might play a large role. Subsequently, knowing what causes fatigue might be influential in determining optimal recovery regimes.

Åstrand and Rodahl (1986) stated that the feeling of fatigue during muscle contractions of high force depends on the blood flow through the muscle. When this is impaired during heavy workloads, the supply of oxygen is compromised as well as the removal of metabolites and heat; this may contribute to short-term loss of function. These various mechanisms as described are likely to play an important role in local muscle fatigue as seen in short, intensive exercise or high force isometric contractions.

The majority of physical activity, however, involves work which incorporates dynamic use of muscles in a continuous repetitive manner; this is characterized as submaximal and involves the generation of relatively low forces which allow for sufficient metabolic recovery between contractions. It appears that central fatigue plays an important role in controlling or limiting performance in prolonged activity. Jones and Round (1990) stated that this occurs due to signals from skin, joint and tendon receptors feeding back to the central nervous system. However, fatigue due to endurance exercise has also been associated with glycogen depletion in the working skeletal muscle (Noakes, 1991). Other factors which contribute to fatigue by affecting central drive and thus motivation include elevated or lowered body core temperature, dehydration, altered blood electrolytes, hypoglycaemia and cerebral hypoxia.

Temperature/thermoregulation

Heat loss and heat production from skeletal muscle is an important homeostatic mechanism for maintenance of core body temperature. Human being are only 20–30% efficient, i.e. only this amount of energy is used in mechanical work while the rest is dissipated as heat. The heat load of exercise or work is dispersed by several heat loss mechanisms, including the evaporative loss from sweating and convective and radiant losses; the magnitude of this loss depends on the temperature and humidity of the working environment. During increasing workloads the core temperature of the body rises; the hypothalamus tries to control this rise using the heat loss mechanisms described above to maintain a heat gradient. It is the dilatation of the skin blood vessels which permits the transfer of heat from the core to the body extremities and outer shell. The mechanism for this vasodilatation is not clearly understood but may be due in part to the activity of sweating and local chemical formation (Edholm and Wiener, 1981).

If protected by clothing, humans can tolerate variations in environmental temperature of between −50°C and +100°C (Åstrand and Rodahl, 1986) but will only tolerate a 4°C increase or 10°C drop in body core temperature without impairment of physical and mental performance. Physical activity can increase the blood flow to the muscle by up to 90%, but in doing so the blood flow to the skin (the peripheral blood flow) will be compromised. Blood has a high capacity to carry a great deal of heat and in heavy exercise this can greatly reduce total endurance capacity because of the need for circulating blood volume to transport heat to the periphery rather than oxygen to the working muscle. Cardiac output is maintained by an increased heart rate but performance is compromised because of a decreased stroke volume. The body, under hypothalamic control, attempts to keep the temperature of the vital organs of brain, heart and gut constant.

If the temperature of the air is lower than the skin then heat loss will occur by radiation and convection and, if the sweat glands are activated, by evaporation. If the environmental temperature is higher than that of the skin (37°C+) then the only means of heat loss is by sweating. The drive to maintain temperature is great and high sweat rates may be achieved, depending on the gradient between the core and shell temperatures. As a person becomes accustomed to heat through the process of acclimatization (Edholm and Wiener, 1981), sweat production increases. Sweating will also occur at an earlier stage during activity, but be more dilute, thus throwing less metabolic load on the tissues from electrolyte loss.

In the workplace, individual differences must be considered, i.e. the elderly worker, the less fit and the obese will have a lowered capacity for acclimatization; women sweat less than men and at a higher core/skin temperature, relying more on circulatory adjustments. It is also important to ensure fluid replacement, particularly in hot, dry temperatures, in order to maintain plasma volume. Fat people should be observed with special care; the specific heat of fat is greater than muscle tissue, thus increasing the insulation and reducing the conduction.

Failure to maintain regulatory control in hot environments may produce heat exhaustion. This is a state of collapse brought on by hypotension which is caused by depletion of plasma volume secondary to sweating and by extreme dilatation of skin blood vessels. In fact, it is a safety valve which ensures cessation of work when heat loss mechanisms are over-taxed. Cold moist skin, dilated pupils and complaints of headaches and giddiness are signs of hypovolaemic shock; rest and intravenous infusion may be needed. If heat exhaustion is not recognized, the more dangerous heat stroke, seen in heatwaves and conditions of hot, still air, may follow; the inability to sweat further causes an inadequate balance of heat loss and gain which can lead to a critical rise in brain temperature (McArdle et al., 1991). Finally, in hot dry environments, especially at altitude, heat cramps in muscles may occur with salt depletion.

Heavy sweat shirts or clothing made of rubber or plastic produce a high relative humidity close to the skin and retard evaporation. If sweat is not allowed to evaporate, cooling is compromised. Likewise, problems may occur if the work rate decreases or if the temperature drops. The person may feel chilled, and cold clammy clothing next to the skin will result in drawing heat from the core and lowering body temperature. Dry clothing also retards heat exchange while clothing which is soaking wet will increase conductivity. Hence it is better for workers in hot temperatures to have loose fitting, light porous clothing which promotes water vapour from the skin.

Human movement at work is a central concern of the physiotherapist in occupational health. The focus should be directed towards encouraging healthy participation in leisure activities to counteract the effects of a sedentary job as well as in protecting the individual from the excessive demands of manual work. The application of physical training theories should be made with judicious regard to the current health status of the individual to ensure a healthy, productive working life.

References

Sports Council and Health Education Authority (1992) *Allied Dunbar National Fitness Survey*, Sports Council, London

Alter, M. J. (1988) *The Science of Stretching*, Human Kinetic Books, Illinois

Åstrand, P. O. and Rodahl, K. (1986) *Textbook of Work Physiology; Physiological Bases of Exercise*, (i) Chapter 8: Evaluation of physical performance on the basis of tests, McGraw–Hill International, Maidenhead

Durnin, J. V. G. A. and Passmore, R. (1967) *Energy, Work and Leisure*, Heinemann, London

Edholm, O. G. and Weiner, J. S. (1981) *Principles and Practice of Human Physiology*, Academic Press, London

Edington, D. W. and Edgerton, V. R. (1976) *The Biology of Physical Activity*, Houghton, Boston

Fentem, P. H., Bassey, E. J. and Turnbull, N. B. (1992) *The New Case for Exercise*, Sports Council and Health Education Authority, London

Huxley, A. F. (1974) *Journal of Physiology*, **243**, 1–43

Jones, D. A. and Round, J. M. (1990) *Skeletal Muscle in Health and Disease, Textbook of Muscle Physiology*, Manchester University Press, Manchester

McArdle, W. D., Katch, F. I. and Katch, V. L. (1991) *Exercise Physiology, Energy, Nutrition and Human Performance*, 3rd edn, Lea and Fabiger, Philadelphia/London

Noakes, T. (1991) *Lore of Running*, Human Kinetics UK, Leeds

Royal College of Physicians of London (1991) *Medical Aspects of Exercise: Benefits and Risks*, Royal College of Physicians, London

Further reading

Brooks, G. A. and Fahey, T. D. (1985) *Exercise Physiology – Human Bioenergetics and its Application*, Macmillan, New York

Chapter 8

Health promotion and education

Barbara Richardson

What is health promotion?

The World Health Organization (WHO) views health promotion as '. . . a unifying concept for those who recognize
the need for change in the ways and conditions of living, in
order to promote better health' (WHO, 1987). The difference
between health promotion and health education is distinguished by Tones et al. (1990). They see health education and
health promotion as having a symbolic relationship. Health
promotion is concerned with building a system which is
conducive to health through health policies which seek to
achieve environmental change and through endeavours
which seek to produce changes in organizations in the
interest of the health of their workers. Health education is an
essential prerequisite of all health promotion programmes
and aims at influencing individual health choices through
enabling critical choices to be made by the individual and
through education of health professionals.

In industrial, business and commercial organizations,
health promotion can be characterized as the provision of a
safe and healthy working environment and of non-harmful
processes and products; health education is the presentation
to people of information on physical, mental and social well-

being which is widely held as likely to maintain or improve their health both now and in later life.

The role of physiotherapy in health promotion and education has been identified only fairly recently in a hospital or community setting (Burkitt, 1986; Lyne, 1986; Norton, 1986). However, in an industrial context, it has been recognized for many years. MacLarty (1986) described a fitness programme which has been offered to the workers of a large retail company through their occupational health services since 1977. Today, the occupational health physiotherapist may be involved in both planning and implementing health promotion programmes and providing the requisite education needed for a successful outcome.

There are many reasons why an organization or an individual health professional in an organization would wish to embark on health promotion. At a national level it may be for the purpose of making savings for the health care and social services of the country, and thus for the taxpayer, or it may be to foster a policy of informed choice, understanding and decision-making by attempting to empower the individual (Tones et al., 1990). In industry, business and commerce it may be done to save the organization money through prevention of occupational injury and related disease, by reducing lost-time injuries and sickness absences and by reducing the likelihood of expensive litigation. Instead, it may be from a commitment to fellow workers to disseminate knowledge which is believed to improve the quality and quantity of their lives.

Before embarking on health promotion in the workplace it is important to consider concepts of health, the relationship between work and health, the ways in which the health goals of individuals in the workplace – management, workers, trade-unionists and health professionals – will differ, and possibly conflict, and one's own feelings on the ethical considerations of getting involved.

Concepts

Sim (1990) gives a useful summary of the principal ways health can be conceptualized and particularly draws attention to the 'disease' model of health which is closely linked to the biomedical perspective of health. He cited Pratt (1989) who argued that physiotherapists work predominantly within a biomedical paradigm in which health is seen only as an absence of disease and affective or cognitive parameters of health are ignored. He pointed out that focusing on biological causes for disease only leads to a 'maintenance' or 'restoration' approach to health and there is no scope for improvement beyond the point of freedom from disease. Health promotion based on this concept of health would thus be aimed exclusively at those who are already unhealthy and would discount the social, cultural and organizational influences on health. Most importantly, 'health' in this concept can be seen as a commodity bestowed on the individual by the health professional, implying a state of dependency rather than a state of being, achievable by the self.

In contrast to the biomedical concept of health, Calnan (1992) looked at some lay concepts of health from a sociological point of view. He cited Blaxter (1990) who conducted a health and lifestyle survey which showed that three different concepts of health were prevalent amongst lay people:

1. A concept of positive fitness, as in the athletic, was most prevalent among men, young people and the better educated.
2. A concept of health as being able to fulfil the social and functional requirements of living was most common in older people.
3. A concept of health based on degrees of not being ill as perceived by the individual was found equally in all social groups, although in females more than men.

The *health belief model*, used to predict compliance of an individual with official health recommended actions, and the *health locus of control theory*, which relates to the perceived autonomy of the individual in taking corrective behaviour, are two theories of health behaviour which further draw attention to the cognitive and affective parameters of health (Calnan, 1992). Looking at health from a sociological point of view in this way can help in providing a clear direction for specific, targeted health education in health promotion programmes. However, such concepts do not define any need to adopt an approach to health other than that of maintenance and restoration.

A more holistic, positive definition of health was put forward by the World Health Organization in 1946 when it stated that: 'Health is a state of complete physical, mental and social well-being and not merely the absence of disease and infirmity'. Whilst commendable for encompassing the contribution to health of all the interacting aspects of life, Sim (1990) argued that this definition portrays health as a Utopian and unattainable status. He put forward more practical concepts of health, such as a capacity to meet demands of the lifestyle of the individual, and further proposed a need to regard health in terms of human potential which embraces all spheres of life in which human aspirations can be realized. He suggested that this concept of health extends beyond the sphere of medical care and may even be incompatible with some aspects of it (see also Owen Hutchinson, 1992).

Being healthy clearly means different things to different people. It is therefore most important for each health professional in the workplace to examine and define for themselves their own concept of health in order to be aware of their own perspective, and then to consider how this relates to health promotion and work.

Relationship between work, health and health promotion

The relationship between work and health is difficult to define. It is argued that the working environment is just one of many factors giving rise to disease and this makes it possible for employers and those in government to focus on aspects, such as personal habits, other than those directly associated with the workplace (French, 1992). In addition, an ongoing debate argues whether unemployment or work is health damaging (Tones et al., 1990). However, the workplace can indisputably be seen as a source of potential hazards including accidents, exposure to substances damaging to health and general work-produced stress, to which the individual would not be exposed if not working and, as such, is worthy of attention by health promoters. The WHO (1987) lists poor physical working conditions, shift work, job overload and underload, role conflict, role insecurity, promotion blockage, two-career families and lack of opportunity for participation in decision making as some work stressors. Manual workers are still considered to be subject to more risk than non-manual workers; they are more likely to be in contact with hazardous substances such as asbestos and coal dust, to be more frequently involved in accidents and to be exposed to high levels of noise. However, Corlett (1983) has also emphasized a need for concern regarding occupational activities which involve static postures as well as dynamic, and Sankaren (1987) has highlighted the attention which needs to be paid to the cervicodorsal region and the arms as a result of the shift of work programmes from the low-back level to the eye level, e.g. work with visual display units and sedentary work.

The Health and Safety at Work Act (Health and Safety Executive, 1974) attempted to ensure safe and healthy working conditions by requiring the provision of education and training programmes which would recognize, avoid and prevent unsafe and unhealthy working conditions by putting responsibility for compliance with the Act on both employer and employee. Response by some employers was apathetic until more specific interpretations were set in place by recent legislation, such as the Reporting of Injury and Dangerous Occurrences Regulations (Health and Safety Executive, 1985), the Control of Substances Hazardous to Health Regulations (Health and Safety Executive, 1988) and the Manual Handling Operations Regulations (Health and Safety Executive, 1992). As a result it can be expected that health protection and health promotion will assume a much higher profile in the workplace, and that organizations will place far more importance on declaring and publishing their policies on the subjects. Within the framework of these Acts and guidelines, management, professionals and workers will all have their own ideas on what needs to be done and what should take priority.

Perspectives of health promotion in the workplace

The many perspectives and expectations of health promotion in the workplace must be acknowledged and acted upon if health promotion programmes are to be successfully accepted by all. Management may judge the worth and success of programmes by economic factors such as increased output and reduced absenteeism, whilst workers are likely to judge them by the perceived improvement to self, commensurate with their ideal of health. Tones et al. (1990) believe that the trade unions will support any initiative which can be shown to be for their members' benefit, 'particularly if executed in "management time"!', but that the workforce in Britain is likely to be more concerned about unemployment than even exposure to hazardous substances, let alone participation in the pursuit of fitness in order to reduce management overheads. Each health professional in the workplace, whether safety officer, or occupational health nurse, hygienist, physiotherapist or doctor, will hold different views of the aims and expectations of health promotion programmes which will reflect their own differing professional goals. It should be unnecessary for fellow workers to feel that their territory is being invaded. The special skills and areas of responsibility of each professional should be clarified and the whole approach to health promotion made by a team and not just one member of staff, who may think she/he is omniscient. Job descriptions should clearly state what is expected of physiotherapists in occupational health. Many are initially employed purely for clinical purposes. However, when faced with opportunities that arise when working in large organizations, it is difficult to ignore the goals of the physiotherapy profession to attempt to educate and prevent the injuries that are treated. When treating a worker with a stiff back or tenosynovitis, most physiotherapists would wish to examine the actual workplace and work posture in an attempt to correct and prevent future occurrences. Is it then ethical to do this for one worker and not for his fellows?

Ethical considerations

The question is raised not only of whose responsibility it is for health promotion, but also the extent of the health promotion proposed. Ideally, if health education were given in the family, the schools and community, encouraged by the government and responsible media, then the role of health promotion in the workplace would appear to be minimal. However within a society which is still comparatively unaccustomed to promoting health, the workplace can be seen as fertile ground for many desirable promotions in addition to those required by the Health and Safety at Work Act. Each health professional must question the right to interfere in fields other than those directly related to the workplace and consider if it is possible to differentiate. As far as physiotherapy is concerned, the whole state of the worker must be taken into consideration, e.g. not simply that the worker's safety shoes are comfortable and safe but also that his/her running shoes are equally satisfactory; not only that the worker knows how to load a lorry, but also that he/she knows how to load the boot of a car.

Other ethical issues question the infringement of people's personal freedom by imposing ideas on them, frightening people by the information given or by the way in which it is presented, and debate whether it is education or indoctrination. Serious thought should also be given to whether we are sure that we are doing the right thing in encouraging measures to be taken to achieve a healthier and longer life 'so that people may live unhappily into their 80s and 90s' (P. Davis, 1993, personal communication). Skrabanek (1990) also pointed out that despite medical experimentation on individuals being controlled by strict ethical guidelines, no protection exists for whole populations which are subject to medical intervention in the name of preventive medicine and health promotion. Such sentiments were succinctly supported by Williams (1984) when she cautioned

'Health promotion like advertising campaigns, cannot hope to do more than induce superficial change which is susceptible to the next round of gimmicks or hard sell. Long-term commitment to sensible health behaviour . . . is needed if we are to improve health, and this is a function of education not promotion. Indeed the very activity of hard-sell promotion is in direct conflict with the rational decision-making and personal autonomy which are central to educational long-term goals and the two cannot co-exist'.

It is clear that health promotion should not be embarked upon lightly and it behoves the occupational health physiotherapist to examine her/his stance on the issues put forward. However, it must be remembered that persuasive techniques to present facts about health hazards or health opportunities in a truthful and balanced way are central to physiotherapy practice and can enhance rather than diminish the autonomy of the individual, since they draw attention to a range of choices of which the individual may not be aware.

Health promotion programmes

Topics

Lifestyle, smoking, drinking, drug abuse, manual handling and lifting, applied ergonomics including avoidance of repetitive strain injury, foot care, stress and relaxation, AIDS and sex education, cancer (well woman and well man clinics), incontinence, sports, training and fitness, pre-employment and pre-retirement, are some of the potential topics for health promotion programmes. The occupational health physiotherapist may be involved as a member or as a leader of a team of health professionals who may be assembled for each programme.

Implementation

Implementation of health programmes in the workplace should involve the following sequence of events:

1. Wait
2. Research
3. Plan
4. Implement
5. Reassess
6. Follow up.

Wait

Health promotion activities should be seen within the framework of an organizational health policy. The support of senior management and the recognized status of the health professional involved are crucial to success. Theory of persuasive communication (Burns, 1991) recognizes that the credibility of the 'source' plays an important part in the reception of the 'message'. It is recommended, therefore, that the occupational health physiotherapist does nothing until in the position long enough to have become well known and to have gained a high reputation and the respect of all (unless, of course, employment has been solely for the purpose of promoting health, but this is likely to be rare). In building this respect and reputation, it is vital to be seen as entirely impartial. The workforce may view the occupational health physiotherapist as an educated professional who wears some badge of office and thus may be considered as associated with management. Whilst attempting to dispel this perception, it is equally important that management does not come to look upon the same person as the worker's champion. It is important, therefore, to attempt to establish a correct rapport at every level of the working hierarchy to enable the accomplishment of professional goals. An initial waiting period gives time to get to know the whole workplace, the people in it and the hierarchy, and to identify areas or workers of particular concern for targeting; it can often lead to more united help and co-operation from everyone involved at a later date.

Research

Having determined the scope and the purpose of a proposed programme, there must be total confidence in the message it will convey. It is important to be able to support ideas with facts and figures which can reach and gain the cooperation of everybody targeted as involved in the programme. The heads of all departments involved should give their approval, including those in occupational health, and particular key figures should be identified, be it the chairman or the workshop foreman, and his/her responsibilities for his/her workforce recognized. Constant referral to management is not 'toadying'. Townsend (1991) put gaining visible senior executive support high on her list of priorities for getting a health and fitness programme operating successfully. Health promotion programmes can cost a lot of money, which must be drawn from the budget of the organization at some level. They may require changes in the working environment or in working practices, may take people away from their jobs for a period of time and will require the occupational health physiotherapist involved to have access to workplaces and/or documents in order to make surveys, monitor implementation and assess outcomes of the programme. It is therefore well within professional interests to ensure appropriate support and cooperation from the start.

Initially, therefore, the research will consist of an approach to the manager/supervisor, to ascertain his reaction to the proposed programme. It is to be hoped that approval and permission to proceed will ensue. The manager's opinion should also be sought as to the time at which the participants will be informed of the proposed programme, and their role in it. The research will then include workplace visits to assess the environment, workstations, operations and activities and attitudes of people who may be targeted. Credibility of the trainer as well as the programme should always be kept in mind. In some circumstances a visiting physiotherapist may be judged by the workforce to be unfamiliar with the content or skills of their work, e.g. dock workers, miners, airfield operators, and all those involved in heavy manual work. In these situations it will be clear that training will be undertaken best through key figures within the working group itself in the workplace. Such potential trainers must be carefully selected for credibility within the group, as well as ability to be trained. Facts and figures on lost-time accidents, sickness absence, etc. should be collated to establish a realistic rationale for the programme. Study of existing legislation, both of the UK and the European Community should be made, as well as company policy and the recommendations of powerful bodies such as the British Standards Institution, the Health and Safety Executive and the Health Education Authority. European Standards should also be taken into consideration. Knowledge of all the regulations may be useful in backing up and substantiating the purpose of a programme, together with clear aims and objectives.

A professional report on the results of the research should be prepared, preferably written and using charts and illustrations for effectiveness where appropriate, and should be given to the necessary level of management for authorization to proceed with the programme and for agreement of the target audience and estimated costs, where available. The report should be as brief as possible and may be presented in *precis* form to senior management, with the full results given to someone lower in the hierarchy or in the technical field. It will subsequently be discussed at the appropriate level and any perceived problems highlighted. These may include:

- Resistance to changes in existing work practices that have been handed down from one generation of worker to another and thus considered infallible.
- Changes in the workplace lay-out and recommendations to supply mechanical aids. Management may well wish to make these alterations before the programme is undertaken.
- Changes in other equipment, e.g. office furniture.
- Union and worker reaction to the proposals, and the potential for stirring up discord or dissatisfaction among the workforce.

Plan

Once approval has been given to proceed, careful planning is essential to ensure success. Pertinent factors to consider are:

- Whether there is a need for a pilot study.
- Is the programme to be held in or out of working hours?
- Mix of participants: managers with workers or separately?; men with women?; all of similar jobs or a mix?
- How best to achieve credibility: run the programme oneself or train supervisors?
- Voluntary or compulsory?
- Theoretical/training department presentation or on-site, or a mixture of both?
- Formal or informal presentation?
- Availability of resources, people and technology.
- Timing – perhaps to coincide with a national promotion.
- Strategies for marketing or advertising the programme: letters, notice boards, house magazines.

Implement

Implementation should be carried out with as much help from the participants as possible, to help establish a sense of identity with and ownership of the programme. They may be asked to be involved with the administration and organization, e.g. reserve the venue, provide visual aids and props, keep attendance records, and, where appropriate, participate in planning and choosing the content of the programme. The manager/supervisor's role in implementation must be recognized and he/she should be encouraged to participate in the programme where appropriate. This will help to emphasize: the importance of the programme and the organization's commitment to it; dispel any feeling of 'them and us' within the workforce; inform the supervisor exactly what the staff are being taught, and thus enable the supervisor to monitor compliance. It may also improve the supervisor's own knowledge of the subject.

The advantages of working with groups as a medium for

disseminating health knowledge are well documented, as are the special communication skills required in group work (Burns, 1991; Ewles and Simnett, 1992). 'People learn best if they are actively involved in the learning process not just passively listening' (Ewles and Simnett, 1992). The age of the lecture, for all practical purposes, is long gone. The workplace has its own special needs in relation to the diverse range of abilities and intellects, belief systems and communication barriers to be found there. A variety of teaching methods appropriate to the adult learner should be employed, involving discussion, group interaction and individual participation, with purposeful use of audio-visual aids (see Newble and Cannon, 1983; Ewles and Simnett, 1992). It is best to work from the known to the unknown: this emphasizes the importance of making a prior assessment of the level of knowledge and capabilities of the target group in order to know where to start. Use of concrete examples and practical problems from the participant's work to illustrate points will ensure relevance.

The change in relationship from the paternalism of the parent/child relationship of the medical model to the contracting and problem-solving adult interaction of mutual support necessary for health promotion activities should not be ignored. 'The mechanisms central to health promotion are self care, or actions that individuals take to enhance their own health and mutual aid, or the actions that people take to support each other' (Scambler, 1991).

Reassess

Reassessment or monitoring of the programme should be part of an ongoing evaluation cycle. Assessment of the post-education state of the workforce should be carried out, feedback obtained and amendments or adjustments to the content or presentation of the programme made where necessary to ensure that objectives are realized. Management interest will be maintained by a formal progress report at regular intervals. The results of any programme should be disseminated as widely as possible to all concerned – managers, participants, helpers – in an appropriate format.

This might be on a notice board or through in-house magazines or, as in the case of one study, informing the local chemist who had agreed to stock 'quit smoking' aids of the success of the programme. In some working groups, prizes may be awarded when no lost-time injuries occur within a specified period, and news of this reported in the in-house journals.

Evaluation

This looks at the programme as a whole, in the light of the aims, and makes a judgement on the outcome and effectiveness of the activity. Evaluation can, and should, be carried out on two levels: outcome and process.

Outcome evaluation can look at changes in knowledge, self awareness or attitudes of the participants through use of interviews, discussion or observation. It can look at changes in behaviour of the participants through demonstration, observation by others or through records of behaviour kept by others. It may also be informative to look for social changes in the organization which may be manifest in policy changes or availability of information, literature or technology. Tones et al. (1990) declared that 'unless conditions appropriate to the adoption of innovations are supplied, an effective workplace programme will not materialise'. It should be recognized that often there will be a time lag before results can be identified and it may be necessary to agree some intermediate indicators of success. This is particularly important when trying to convince management of a positive outcome.

Process evaluation looks at the method used to execute the programme. Evaluation can be made by self-evaluation, peer evaluation (the opinions of other informed professionals), or client evaluation (the opinions of the workers, managers or supervisors).

Careful scrutiny of the results of evaluation should allow planning for the future. The results might indicate a need to target more specifically, include other areas of knowledge or information, scale down objectives to a more realistic, achievable level or change the method of evaluation itself. It is important to document and record such evaluations and aim where possible to share experiences with others through discussion or publishing.

Follow-ups and refreshers

It is sometimes beneficial to follow up a programme at a later date with a formal or informal assessment. Sometimes it will be necessary to recommend refresher programmes as a consequence, if not already in place. In carrying out such programmes and considering further programmes there is a need to beware of overkill, of getting a reputation for snooping in the workplace or being seen as a 'quasi-secret services man'. Promoting health successfully in an organization over the long term depends a great deal upon working sensitively and intuitively with all levels of the workforce.

Future developments

Adoption of a *health career approach* to individuals in organizations, as well as to individuals, is beginning to emerge (Tones *et al.*, 1990). In this approach appropriate teaching is given at specific points in the health career of an individual at work. The same topics are taught to the same individuals at intervals and re-presented in ways which are meaningful for that age or stage of development of disease. In keeping with this are *employment assistance programmes*. These employ health and fitness initiatives with training and counselling (Lamport Mitchell, 1991), and aim to provide mechanisms to increase the chances for continued employment of individuals whose job performance may be threatened by individual problems of a physical or mental nature. Other similar schemes are developing in Scandinavia with regard to the ageing worker (Korhonen, 1988). Confidentiality, commitment and a conviction by the workforce that admitting to problems, whether of alcohol or arthritis, will not lead to job loss, is paramount to the success of these programmes.

It is believed that health promotion programmes may offer disease prevention and health protection which can produce behaviour change, reduce risks and reduce costs in an organization. There is a continuing need for carefully-designed research of these programmes to confirm this belief. Many indicators of the success of workplace programmes are long term and should be realized by changes in organizational philosophy and policies or by provision of appropriate technology, as well as changes in worker behaviour. To have any enduring effect, health promotion programmes should become part of the culture of an organization. The physiotherapist in occupational health can and should play a full part in achieving this goal.

Acknowledgement

I should like to acknowledge the considerable assistance of Miss Prue Davis (former occupational health physiotherapist with Shell UK Ltd) in preparing this chapter.

References

Blaxter, M. (1990) *Health and Lifestyles*, Routledge, London

Burkitt, A. (1986) Health, health education and the physiotherapist. *Physiotherapy*, **72**, 2–4

Burns, R.R. (1991) *Essential Psychology*, 2nd edn, Kluwer Academic Publishers and MTP Press, Lancaster, p. 236 and p. 238

Calnan, M. (1992) Lay beliefs about health and illness. In *Physiotherapy: A Psychosocial Approach* (ed. S. French), Butterworth–Heinemann, Oxford

Corlett, E.N. (1983) Analysis and evaluation of working posture. In *Ergonomics of Workstation Design* (ed. T.O. Kvålseth), Butterworth, London

Ewles, L. and Simnett, L. (1992) *Promoting Health, A Practical Guide to Health Education*, 2nd edn, John Wiley, Chichester

French, S. (1992) Inequalities in health. In *Physiotherapy, A Psychosocial Approach* (ed. S. French), Butterworth–Heinemann, Oxford

Health and Safety Executive (1974) *Health and Safety at Work Act*, HMSO, London

Health and Safety Executive (1985) *The Reporting of Injury and Dangerous Occurrences Regulations*, HMSO, London

Health and Safety Executive (1988) *Control of Substances Hazardous to Health Regulations*, HMSO, London

Health and Safety Executive (1992) *Manual Handling Operations Regulations*, HMSO, London

Korhonen, T. (1988) Taking a break improves performance. In *Work Health Safety 1988*, Institute of Occupational Health, Helsinki, Finland

Lamport Mitchell J. (1991) Stress in life and work. *Occupational Health*, **43**, 19–20

Lyne, P. A. (1986) The professions allied to medicine – their potential contribution to health education. *Physiotherapy*, **72**, 8–10

MacLarty, J. (1986) The fitness programme at Marks and Spencer head office. *Physiotherapy*, **72**, 54–56

Newble, D. and Cannon, R. (1983) *A Handbook for Clinical Teachers*, MTP Press, Lancaster

Norton, S. (1986) Support for physiotherapists in health education. *Physiotherapy*, **72**, 5–7

Owen Hutchinson, J. S. (1992) Health, health education and physiotherapy practice. In *Physiotherapy: A Psychosocial Approach* (ed. S. French), Butterworth–Heinemann, Oxford

Pratt, J. W. (1989) Towards a philosophy of physiotherapy. *Physiotherapy*, **75**, 114–120

Sankaren, B. (1987) Musculoskeletal injuries in the workplace. *Ergonomics*, **30**, 465–467

Scambler, G. (1991) *Sociology as Applied to Medicine*, 3rd edn, Baillière Tindall, London

Sim, J. (1990) The concept of health. *Physiotherapy*, **76**, 423–427

Skrabanek, P. (1990) Why is preventive medicine exempted from ethical constraints? *Journal of Medical Ethics*, **16**, 187–190

Tones, K, Tilford, S. and Robinson, Y. (1990) *Health Education, Effectiveness and Efficiency*, Chapman and Hall, London

Townsend, J. (1991) Making health and fitness promotion work. *Occupational Health*, **43**, 14–15

Williams, G. (1984) Health promotion – caring concern or slick salesmanship? *Journal of Medical Ethics*, **10**, 191–195

World Health Organization (1946) *Constitution of the World Health Organization*, WHO, Geneva

World Health Organization (1987) *Health Promotion in the Working World*. Report on a joint meeting organized by the Federal Centre for Health Education (Cologne, 1985) WHO, Copenhagen

Further reading

Adams, C. and Tidyman, M. (1987) *Give Up For Good*, National Extension College, Cambridge

Batten, L. and Allen, S. (1991) *Towards A Smoke Free Environment*, Health Education Authority, London

Cooper, C. L. and Payne, R. (1991) Individual differences in health behaviour. In *Personality and Stress: Individual Differences in the Stress Process*, Ch. 10, John Wiley, Chichester

Cranfield, S. and Dixon, A. (1990) *HIV and AIDS in the 1990s – A Guide for Training Professionals*, Health Education Authority, London

Downie, R. S., Fyfe, C. and Tannahill, A. (1992) *Health Promotion, Models and Values*, Oxford Medical Publications, Oxford

Hardy, C. (1991) *Swimming for Health*, Hodder and Stoughton, London

Heller, T., Bailey, L. and Pattison, S. (1992) *Preventing Cancer*, Oxford University Press, Oxford

Heron, J. (1989) *The Facilitator's Handbook*, Kogan Page, London

Jenkins, M. and McEwen, J. (1988) *Smoking Policies at Work*, Cambridge University Press, Cambridge

Mitchell, L. (1988) *Simple Relaxation*, John Murray, London

Secretary of State (1992) *Health Of The Nation*, HMSO, London

Steele, C. (1990) *Smoker's Quit Plan*, Gardiner–Caldwell Communications, Macclesfield

Tether, P. and Robinson, D. (1986) *Preventing Alcohol Problems*, Tavistock Publications, London

Trent, D. R. (1991) *Promoting Mental Health*, vol. 1, Avebury, Aldershot

Useful addresses

British Heart Foundation, 102 Gloucester Place, London W1H 4DH

Health Education Authority, Hamilton House, Mabledon Place, London WC1

National Back Pain Association, 31–33 Park Rd., Teddington, Middlesex TW11 0AB

Chapter 9

Fitness and health programmes

Christopher Norris

Nature of modern-day disease

The nature of disease in Britain has changed considerably over the last century. At one time a combination of poverty, deficient diet and inadequate sanitation bred infectious diseases. Nowadays, however, affluence has brought an over-indulgent lifestyle and a whole catalogue of chronic ailments. As a result, typhoid and TB have given way to heart disease and cancer as the major causes of premature disability in our society. However, rather than being problems of old age, these current diseases often ravage those who are still young and productive. The result carries a heavy price. It has been estimated that coronary heart disease (CHD) cost the nation over £1 billion in 1985, with 50 million working days being lost as a direct result of cigarette smoking (Ashton, 1990). The purpose of a fitness and health programme is to confront this modern epidemic and give employees the chance to fight back.

Risk factors

The corporate fitness centre should be part of an overall health promotion strategy which addresses the various risk

Table 9.1 Risk factors

Coronary heart disease
Smoking
High fat diet
High triglyceride levels (high LDL, low HDL)
High blood pressure
Physical inactivity
Obesity
Diabetes (especially with onset before age 40)
Inability to cope with stress
Coronary-prone personality
Family history of coronary heart disease or stroke
Low back pain
Inadequate trunk muscle endurance
Inadequate leg muscle endurance
Lack of flexibility in midtrunk and hamstrings
Poor posture
Faulty body mechanics
Poor ability in lifting techniques
Low cardiopulmonary fitness levels

LDL, low density lipoprotein; HDL, high density lipoprotein.

factors associated with disease, especially CHD. Risk factors for CHD and low back pain are shown in Table 9.1. The corporate fitness centre can act as the hub of a more general health promotion programme aimed at reducing the risk of disease in the workforce. General health screening (see below), dietary advice and weight reduction, smoking cessation, stress control and relaxation training must all be addressed.

Health benefits of exercise

A full discussion of the benefits of exercise is outside the scope of this chapter, but some understanding of the useful adaptations to be gained from regular exercise will help the occupational health physiotherapist argue the case for exercise as part of a health care programme. Some of the benefits of regular exercise are listed in Table 9.2. For further details the reader is referred to the Further reading list at the end of the chapter.

Musculoskeletal disorders

The use of exercise in the management of musculoskeletal disorders is widespread in physiotherapy. The preventive benefits of exercise in terms of musculoskeletal stress and injury are less accepted. Certainly, some musculoskeletal back pain may result from postural changes which can be reversed by exercise (McKenzie, 1981; Cailliet, 1983; Dimaggio and Mooney, 1987). Reflex weakening of muscle occurs following injury and pain (de Andrade et al., 1965; Stokes and Young, 1984), and restoration of strength and flexibility is important following any musculoskeletal injury if problems are not to recur. Poor condition of the trunk muscles has been identified as an important factor in back injury prevention (Richardson et al., 1992).

Correcting faulty movement patterns is equally important to the total restoration of function. A reduction in the number and variety of movements to which the body is subjected has been suggested as one causal factor in musculoskeletal injury (Janda, 1992). It is likely that a reduction in any, or all, of the components of fitness may make musculoskeletal injury more likely. Strength and flexibility decrements have been associated with increased numbers of sports injuries (Renstrom and Kannus, 1992) and enhancement of cardiopulmonary fitness has been shown to reduce the likelihood of back pain (Cady et al., 1979; Kellett et al., 1991). A reduction in skill (especially balance and co-ordination ability) is also likely to increase the likelihood of injury in the industrial work situation. The implementation of a physical training programme to increase endurance time of repetitive tasks has been used with some success (Asfour et al., 1984; Genaidy et al., 1989; Genaidy et al., 1990).

The use of functional screening of the musculoskeletal system has been recommended as a preventive measure for musculoskeletal injury, especially back pain (Lewit, 1991). Testing muscular endurance of the back muscles has been

Table 9.2 Links between the physiological improvements attributable to exercise and their favourable effects on the natural history of disease and degenerative conditions

Physiological improvement	'Prevention'/amelioration of disease
Functions which can be enhanced by regular exercise:	Thus exercise:
Cardiovascular function	
Cardiac performance/ myocardial work	• Ameliorates the effects of age and chronic disease (including CVD),
Arterial blood pressure regulation	• Reduces BP in mild hypertension; attenuates age-dependent rise in BP
Cardiovascular and sympatho-adrenal response to acute exercise	• Reduces risk of cardiac arrhythmias and possibly of sudden death
Electrical stability of heart muscle	
Skeletal muscle	
Metabolic capacities	• Ameliorates effects of age
Nutrient blood supply	and chronic disease on
Contractile properties	reserve capacity for exercise, increasing endurance and reducing fatigue
Strength	• Reduces risk of injury; ameliorates effects of muscle disease
Tendons and connective tissues	
Strength	• Reduces risk of injury,
Supportive function	especially with age and
Increase joint stability	muscle disease
Skeleton	
Maintenance of bone mass and adjustment of structure to load	• 'Prevents' osteoporosis and fractures
Joints	
Lubrication	• Avoids limitation of movements
Range of movement	• Limits effects of degenerative
Maintenance of flexiblity	arthritis

Table 9.2 (*Continued*)

Physiological improvement	'Prevention'/amelioration of disease
Metabolic function	
Body weight control; regulation of energy balance	• 'Prevents' obesity-related disease and excessive weight gain
Carbohydrate tolerance	• Improves carbohydrate tolerance; ameliorates late-onset diabetes
Lipid and lipoprotein metabolism	• 'Prevents' coronary vessel disease
Inhibition of blood clotting processes and platelet aggregation	• Counters acute precipitants of 'heart attack'
Psychological function	
Mood	• Reduces mild anxiety and depression
Self-esteem	• Influences mood favourably
Psychomotor development	• Contributes to quality of care for the mentally handicapped
Memory	• Improves memory in the elderly
Stress reduction	• Ameliorates stress-related conditions

CVD, cerebrovascular disease; BP, blood pressure. From Fentem, 1992.

shown to be an accurate predictor of the likelihood of developing back pain (Biering-Sørensen, 1984). Musculoskeletal pain is a condition which has a multifactorial aetiology, and it seems likely that the various components of physical fitness are important co-factors.

Additional benefits to a company

In addition to the direct health benefits of exercise, a corporate fitness centre offers many other indirect benefits to a company in terms of work performance, absenteeism, job satisfaction, recruitment and company image. An employee who is fitter may be more efficient and achieve a greater productivity level. An association exists between participation in a corporate fitness programme and absenteeism (Donoghue, 1977; Bowne et al. 1984, Baun et al., 1986). However, whether the association is causal is not certain. Certainly, it is easy to think that an employee who is more physically fit may be less likely to suffer from illness resulting in absenteeism. However, a certain amount of self-selection exists whereby employees who tend to join a fitness scheme may be the type who have less absence anyway. Actual participation in a corporate fitness programme on a regular basis has been shown to give a greater positive change in work attendance (Lynch et al., 1990) but the reason for this change could be attributed to the physiological benefits of exercise or more general social and psychological factors.

Participation in a corporate fitness programme can improve job satisfaction. Exercise has been shown to enhance self-confidence, self-esteem and body image (Vincent, 1976; Sonstroem, 1984) and reductions in anxiety, depression, stress and tension have also been demonstrated (Cooper, 1982). Reductions in stress and anxiety have been reported lasting 2–5 hours after the cessation of training (Morgan, 1985), and weight training programmes have been shown to enhance self-concept in male participants (Dishman and Gettman, 1981; Tucker, 1982) as well as female ones (Brown and Harrison, 1986). Employee attitudes have been shown to change positively following participation in a health promotion programme (Holzbach et al., 1990). Significant changes in attitudes to organizational commitment, working conditions, pay and fringe benefits, and job security were noted.

Establishing a corporate fitness centre can enhance company image and may make job recruitment easier. An individual interested in health and fitness may favour a company which offers such facilities (Ashton, 1989). In addition, this type of individual is likely to place a high value on health and fitness facilities. This can be an important factor when thinking of moving to another company and may result in a reduction in staff turnover.

Because employees exercise in a corporate fitness centre together, the facility can enhance group cohesion and teambuilding. Employees get the opportunity to meet others from all levels of the company. This can make those higher up in a company seem less remote and enable managers to relate more easily to staff.

Exercise type and quantity

In order to produce a training effect, the body must be worked harder by exercise than it would be during everyday activities. To do this an overload stimulus is required. In general, the greater the overload the greater the training effect. However, there is a minimum amount of activity required to produce a training effect capable of improving health. Similarly, an overload which is too great may have an adverse effect on the body, giving rise to a greater number of injuries and reducing the effectiveness of the immune system (Nieman and Nehlsen-Cannarella, 1992). The correct frequency, intensity and duration of training is therefore essential. The American College of Sports Medicine (ACSM, 1978) recommended the quantity and quality of exercise required to develop and maintain aerobic fitness and body composition. A training frequency of 3–5 days per week is required, at an intensity of 60–90% maximum heart rate reserve or 50–85% maximal oxygen uptake ($\dot{V}O_2$max). This should be carried out for a duration of 15–60 min, and be continuous and rhythmical in nature. These recommendations were later updated (ACSM, 1990) to include the provision of resistance training sufficient to develop and maintain fat-free weight in the adult. One set of eight to 12 repetitions of between eight and ten exercises that condition the major muscle groups should be used at least twice each week.

Specialist bodybuilding programmes should be generally avoided in the corporate fitness setting, as they concentrate on strength alone and do not give a balanced fitness programme. In addition, they may reduce flexibility and lead to postural imbalances. Programmes which last longer than 60 min per training session tend to have higher dropout rates than shorter exercise periods (Pollock, 1988).

An exercise programme should generally begin with a warm-up period designed to induce mild sweating and take the major joints through their full range of notion. The main part of the exercise programme should involve the major muscle groups and be controlled and rhythmical in nature. Examples of exercise types include circuit weight training, aerobic dance and callanetics. At the end of the exercise period a cool down should be performed to allow the body to return to resting levels slowly.

Fitness facilities

Once an organization recognizes the benefits of exercise, the method used to bring about these benefits must be decided. Various approaches may be taken depending on the commitment of the company and the finances available (Table 9.3). In its simplest form, activity may be encouraged by supporting the formation of sports clubs and sections outside working hours. Football and running clubs, for example, can be identified with the company through the use of the company logo on sportswear. Reduced membership fees may be negotiated at local council- or privately- run health clubs. Exercise tapes or videos may be purchased for use in a casual aerobics class in the dinner hour or after work.

This type of involvement in exercise promotion is very low cost, but tends to encourage the individual who is already participating in exercise simply to change venue. One of the main aims of a corporate fitness centre is to improve the overall health of the workforce. To achieve this, those individuals who are in the high-risk group for CHD must be encouraged to participate in controlled exercise. Therefore a major target market for the corporate fitness centre is the individual who does not exercise regularly, and often sees no reason to do so. To be of benefit to these individuals and to ensure the provision of safe exercise, the corporate fitness facility must be seen as part of the medical, rather than recreational, facilities of a company.

To encourage the less motivated individual to exercise, a fitness programme must be convenient. An on-site facility is likely to achieve better compliance. It should provide an

Table 9.3   Fitness facilities

Level one
Shower cubicle in toilet block
Walk/jogging route
Exercise tape/video in large room or corridor
Encourage use of local leisure centres, block booking and/or
    reduced fees
Literature on health factors at key points

Level two
As above plus:
    Room with exercise cycles
    Exercise teacher to take aerobics class
    Blood pressure monitoring and health questionnaire by nurse

Level three
Separate changing and showering facilities
Small on-site gymnasium with multigym unit and exercise cycles
Exercise classes with teacher
Sessional physiotherapist for basic fitness/health screening and
    exercise prescription to unfit employees; basic rehabilitation
    and treatment

Level four
Full on-site corporate fitness facility
Comprehensive health and fitness screening including resting
    ECG
Sessional or full-time physiotherapist for rehabilitation and
    treatment service
Health promotion service

Level five
Full on-site facilities including gym, sauna and pool, squash
    courts
Full-time physiotherapist
Health screening, fitness testing and treadmill ECG under
    medical supervision
Full health promotion including well woman and well man

ECG, electrocardiogram.

appealing environment in which to exercise, with clean
changing and showering facilities, user-friendly apparatus, a
convenient location, suitable staffing and good programme
administration.

The room chosen should have easy access, with good car parking, and be on a commonly used route, for example near the staff restaurant. The facility should provide separate male and female changing rooms of the type found in a top class leisure complex. Individual cubicles and lockers are generally preferred by self-conscious individuals.

The equipment chosen should aim at improving cardiopulmonary fitness and be suitable for basic muscle toning and bodyshaping. Examples of cardiopulmonary apparatus include static cycles, running machines (treadmills), rowing machines, step climbers, skiing machines and rebounders. Weight training apparatus is used for muscle toning, and can be used to maintain cardiopulmonary fitness (Gettman et al., 1978). The type of apparatus chosen must reflect the nature of the corporate fitness centre as a fitness, rather than competitive sporting, facility. Apparatus should be safe and effective, convenient to use and visually appealing. Multistack weight training apparatus is probably more suitable, and various types are available (Table 9.4). Weight training apparatus and technique has been detailed elsewhere (Norris, 1993).

Small apparatus such as skipping ropes, light dumbbells, flexibands and ankle weights can be used to introduce variety into an exercise programme. The use of mirrors helps with exercise technique and the environment itself should be appealing, with music, plants, carpeting, pastel shades of decor and instructional posters and charts.

Health evaluation

Health evaluation or 'screening' has a number of important functions (Howley and Franks, 1986). First, it may be used to establish if an employee has a history of any relevant medical problems. Second, any signs and symptoms which may indicate underlying health problems can be recorded. Third, health risk factors may be identified and behavioural traits associated with health can be catalogued. An additional function of health evaluation is to use the test results as

Table 9.4 Checklist for selecting exercise equipment

Ease of operation
Is the apparatus self explanatory?
Can the weight be adjusted from the exercising position?
Are the pulleys and weights smooth in operation?
Is the machine comfortable to use?
Can the machine be adjusted to suit a wide variety of users?

Durability
Is the machine construction suited to heavy corporate usage?
Can the machine be cleaned easily?
What is the machine's recommended life?

Safety
Are all moving parts enclosed?
Can fingers/limbs be trapped easily if the machine is used
  incorrectly?
Is the machine stable?
Does the unit pass the current safety standards?

Aesthetics
Is the unit visually appealing?
Is the appearance of the machine daunting to novice users?
Will the machine appeal to a wide range of users?

Support and documentation
What is the guarantee period on the unit?
Is a maintenance contract included or available?
What is the call-out period for maintenance?
Is a well presented user's manual included?

Company reputation
Does the manufacturer have a good reputation?
How long has the manufacturer been in business?
What is the financial position of the company?

Biomechanical suitability
Is the machine based on sound biomechanical principles?
Is the unit designed correctly for the body part to be exercised?
Are the minimum starting weights and weight increments
  suitable for rehabilitation usage?

Adapted from Storlie et al., 1992.

motivators for lifestyle changes which address any identified
risk factors.

Screening can vary, from the use of simple questionnaires designed to give an employee a quantifiable score of his or her risk factors, to full clinical tests of the cardiopulmonary system. A full medical questionnaire is normally completed and various biometric measurements are taken, such as blood pressure, body fat, height and weight, lung capacity and blood lipids. Behavioural variables such as activity and exercise habits, smoking, alcohol usage and diet are assessed. A 'stress questionnaire' may be used relating to recent changes in life/home situation and attitudinal variables such as general well-being, self image, job satisfaction and relationships with fellow workers.

From the initial subjective assessment and basic biometric tests, employees are classified as low or high cardiopulmonary risk. Those at low risk may proceed to a fitness test and exercise programme while being continually monitored by the occupational health physiotherapist. The high-risk employees should be referred to the occupational health physician who can then decide if the employee should be investigated by a cardiologist, or alternatively, is safe to proceed to the exercise programme. All employees, whether low or high risk, may receive a health education programme. High-risk employees may require a weight loss programme and medication to control other risk factors such as hypertension and hyperlipidaemia before proceedings to a modified exercise programme.

An exercise test may be used to determine fitness level expressed as predicted $\dot{V}O_2max$ using cycle ergometry or a more simple step test. Treadmill testing may be used for both fitness testing and clinical evaluation of cardiopulmonary variables. Field tests may be utilized for strength and flexibility, and physiotherapy evaluation used to assess the musculoskeletal system.

Periodic reassessments are performed to monitor progress and maintain employee motivation. Reassessments may be performed as regularly as every 2–4 weeks for very unfit employees. Not all tests are performed, but the idea is to show the employee that some progress is being made to maintain his or her motivation. Well motivated employees, especially athletes, will only need reassessments every 6–12 months; they do not require the same level of individual attention as the unfit individual and their interest in the scheme can be more easily maintained through promotional events.

Running the scheme

Staffing

For a corporate fitness centre to run safely and effectively, some degree of supervision is necessary. Corporate fitness staff have a number of functions. They can prescribe exercise programmes, motivate employees, and have an administrative function which may also include promoting the centre within the company. If the centre is to run effectively, one of the staff members should be a chartered physiotherapist. This is because a large proportion of the centre users will be unfit adults, and as such may already be suffering from clinical conditions which can be easily exacerbated by incorrectly prescribed or poorly executed exercise. Such conditions typically include back pain, chronic soft tissue injuries and cardiopulmonary problems. However, it is essential that the chartered physiotherapist update his or her knowledge of exercise with additional study in a sports science discipline which includes exercise physiology, biomechanics and sports psychology.

There is sometimes a tendency for companies to want unsupervised fitness centres which may simply have a number of instructional wall posters. This type of facility lacks precise exercise prescription and leadership, and employees quickly lose motivation to attend. A centre of this type rapidly becomes a poorly attended recreational facility attracting individuals who would normally use the local sports centre.

Management of the scheme can be carried out by an administrator (who may also be a physiotherapist or nurse with management training). It is their function to oversee the everyday running of the centre, and to administer any promotions which may be run.

Local exercise teachers can be recruited to run classes such as aerobics and yoga. If the exercise specialist in charge of the scheme had the expertise to run these, it may still be better to get an outside tutor, as a 'change of face' can often motivate people to attend. Classes involving employees of low fitness levels should be taught by a physiotherapist. Once an employee's fitness level has improved sufficiently they may be transferred to another class. Similarly, contractors may be used for health promotion classes such as smoking cessation, weight watching and relaxation courses. It is important that the physiotherapist in charge of the corporate fitness centre keeps a tight rein on classes run by external agencies, to ensure standards of professionalism and class content.

Ensuring participant adherence

To continue to gain benefit from the corporate fitness centre, employees must exercise regularly. Unfortunately many individuals start with good intentions, but then typically about half will stop coming (Franklin, 1984). Ensuring that employees continue to use the fitness facilities is an important leadership challenge for fitness centre staff, and involves a basic understanding of client motivation techniques.

Factors which act as motivation will fulfil a 'need' in the employee and these needs will continually change. For example, one of the needs may be to lose several inches from around the waist. This will not be as large a motivating factor in the week before Christmas as it is in the week before the employee's summer holiday on a beach. Consequently, the first stage in the motivation process should be to assess an employee's needs during a one-to-one consultation.

Having identified the needs, these must be acted on and a motivator chosen. This will normally be a combination of both intrinsic and extrinsic factors. Intrinsic motivators rely on a client's feelings and are personal to them, while extrinsic motivators rely on something external such as a prize or trophy. One effective form of motivation is goal setting. A goal may be either long- or short-term, but must be specific. For example, it is more effective to encourage an employee to try to run a certain distance and time on a treadmill by a particular date rather than simply trying to 'improve'. At the same time, a goal must stretch the employees if it is to give them something to aim at, but not be so difficult that it is out of their reach. Goals are set individually, and it is often helpful to have a form printed which the employee signs and dates as a symbol of commitment.

Promotional activities (Table 9.5) are used to maintain a high profile for the fitness centre. A calender of events should be drawn up to plan the whole year (Figure 9.1). Events may be linked with specific periods such as Easter and Christmas, or to dates such as Valentine's day and bonfire night. Seasonal events for body toning before the summer holidays and weight loss in the new year are normally popular. Workshops on common sports such as tennis and jogging may be linked to media coverage of Wimbledon and the London marathon, for example.

Showing success can be an important method of fitness centre promotion. Featuring employees in the company newspaper who have reached specific targets with weight loss, body fat or body measurements, for example, can be successful providing their permission is sought first. This type of coverage will usually have the effect of motivating others, who may think 'if they can do it, so can I'.

A single sponsored charity event can be highly successful and has a number of advantages. Specific employees can be given the responsibility of organizing the event. This has a knock-on effect of developing project management and man management skills in these individuals. The event can be organized through departments to instigate a teambuilding process. The event itself runs for a defined timescale and gradually builds interest as it grows. When a pre-determined target is achieved, a senior executive in the company should then present the cheque to charity with the individuals who organized the event. This gives recognition to the efforts of all involved, and provides positive local media coverage for the company.

Table 9.5 Promotional activities

Newsletter produced on a desk-top publishing system, to include articles on health and fitness and features on employees who have been successful in losing weight, etc.

Health fair stands on health and fitness topics, e.g. blood pressure and body fat measuring; demonstrations on cooking and nutritional content of food; measurement of lung capacity; heart rate monitoring on static cycles

Electronic mail. Use of company E-mail system to announce future events and keep a running timetable of activities

Posters produced in house or bought in. Competitions for best logo or feature, etc.

Flyers. Handouts featuring single fitness events to hand out or include in wage packets

Display boards featuring a single theme such as back pain, accompanied by posters and leaflets. Display moved around the site, spending 1 week in each department

Canteen table displays advertising health events

Single seminars and videos aimed at particular target markets, e.g. 'back pain and gardening'

Courses limited to 4–6 sessions only, developing specific aspects of fitness, e.g. 'jogging for fun'; 'tummy toning'

Workout classes. Ongoing, such as aerobics, step, circuit training, stretch and relax

Incentive and awards system. Different coloured tee shirts after 10, 20, 50 workouts. Prizes when set goals are achieved. Gym member of the month. Gold award for achievement

Buddy system. Once instructed to use the gym, an employee exercises with a training partner with similar aims who has been using the gym for some time

Goal setting. Goals agreed at time of physical assessment, on performance or physical measurements such as body fat and weight loss

Exercise trail. Jogging trail with exercise stations to perform simple callanetics, mobility and balance

Table 9.5 (*Continued*)

Computer self-assessment. Testing an employee's knowledge of healthy lifestyle, for example

Fitness challenge. Points gained for attendance at certain events or performing exercise off-site. Winner achieves set number of points first

Sponsored events, e.g. 24-hour sponsored static cycle ride; Land's End to John O'Groats run on treadmills; total 500 hours of exercising, graphing progress in the gym

Fun run, usually as a conclusion of other event such as health fare or fitness challenge, involving the whole family. Prizes for different age groups

Quiz on nutrition or lifestyle to involve Company and family members together in teams

---

Evaluating the scheme

One important question we must be able to answer is: 'Does it work?'. Continual monitoring of standards and effectiveness enables us to carry on justifying the centre and to argue for greater funding in the future.

Three factors should be considered: outcome, impact and process evaluation (Storlie et al., 1992). Outcome evaluation looks at the results which were achieved. For example, was there a reduction in average blood pressure, or a general decline in body weight of centre participants? Such physiological variables are readily available from fitness assessments and may be used to compare the effectiveness of various schemes over a period of time. For example, was average weight loss greater from weight training programmes or aerobics classes? Impact evaluation measures how behaviour and attitude were affected by the scheme. Assessment is generally made by questionnaires completed before attending the fitness centre and after exercising for a certain period. Process evaluation looks at qualitative aspects of programme delivery in terms of participant satisfaction. For example, which teaching methods are better liked when instructing in the gym?

Statistics must be gathered periodically. These may be

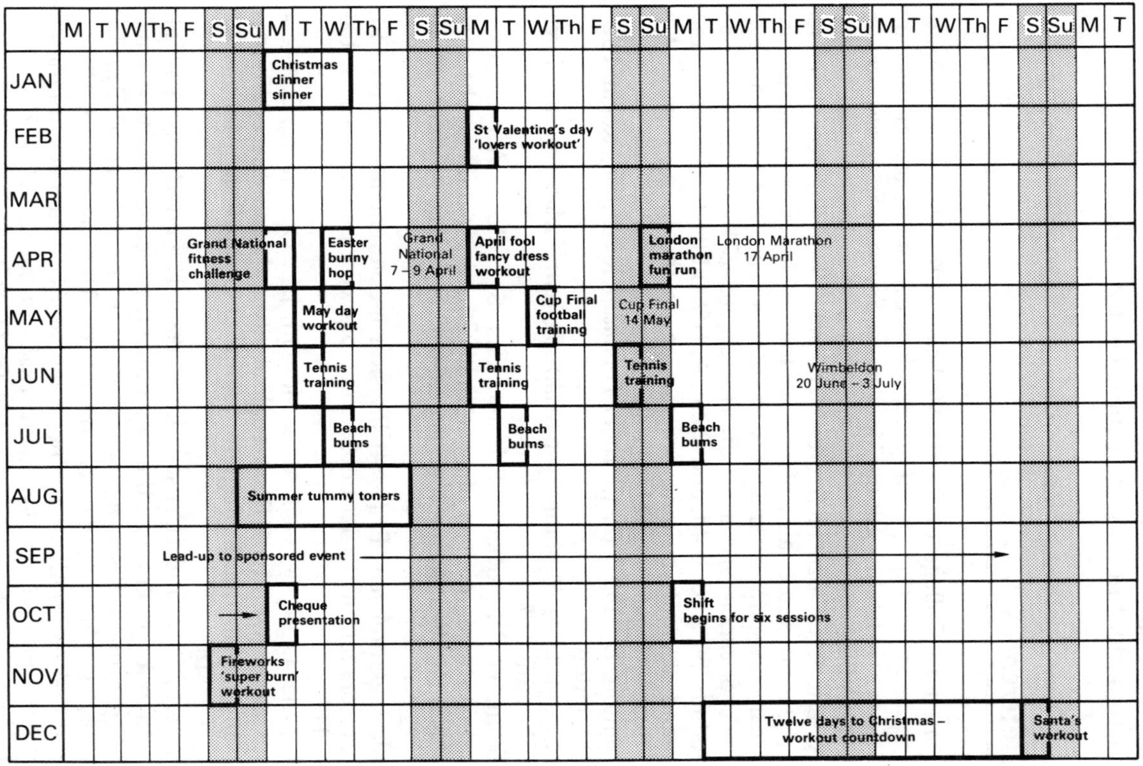

Fig. 9.1 Calendar of fitness events.

monthly, quarterly or annual, and summarize centre
utilization (total numbers in each scheme, age and sex
distribution, regularity of attendance) as well as other
factors identified by the fitness centre staff.

References

American College of Sports Medicine (1978) The recommended
quantity and quality of exercise for developing and maintaining
fitness in healthy adults. *Medicine and Science in Sports and Exercise*,
10, VII–X

American College of Sports Medicine (1990) The recommended
quantity and quality of exercise for developing and maintaining
cardiorespiratory and muscular fitness in healthy adults. *Medicine
and Science in Sports and Exercise*, **22**, 265–274

Asfour, S., Ayoub, M. and Mital, A. (1984) Effects of an endurance
and strength training programme on the lifting capability of
males. *Ergonomics*, **27**, 435–442

Ashton, D. (1989) *The Corporate Healthcare Revolution*, Kogan Page,
London

Ashton, D. (1990) Employee health. *Personnel Management*, March,
factsheet 27

Baun, W. B., Bernacki, E. J. and Tsai, S. P. (1986) A preliminary
investigation: effect of a corporate fitness program on absenteeism and health care cost. *Journal of Occupational Medicine*, **28**, 18–
22.

Biering-Sørensen, F. (1984) Physical measurements as risk indicators for low back trouble over a one year period. *Spine*, **9**, 106–
119

Bowne, D. W., Russell, M. L. Morgan, J. L. Optenberg, S. A. and
Clarke, A. E. (1984) Reduced disability and health, care costs in an
industrial fitness program. *Journal of Occupational Medicine*, **26**,
809–816

Brown, R. D. and Harrison, J. M. (1986) The effects of a strength
training program on the strength and self-concept of two female
age groups. *Research Quarterly for Exercise and Sport*, **57**, 315–320

Cady, L., Bischoff, D., O'Connell, E., Thomas, P. and Allan, J.
(1979) Strength and fitness and subsequent back injuries in
firefighters. *Journal of Occupational Medicine*, **21**, 269–272

Cailliet, R. (1983) *Soft Tissue Pain and Disability*, FA Davis, Philadelphia

Cooper, K. H. (1982) *The Aerobics Programme for Total Well-being*, Bantam publishers, New York

de Andrade, J. R., Grant, C. and Dixon, A. (1965) Joint distension and reflex muscle inhibition in the knee. *Journal of Bone and Joint Surgery*, **47**, 313–322

Dimaggio, A. and Mooney, V. (1987) The McKenzie program: exercise effective against back pain. *Journal of Musculoskeletal Medicine*, **4**, 63–74

Dishman, R. K. and Gettmen, L. R. (1981) Psychological vigour and self-perceptions of increased strength. *Medicine and Science in Sports and Exercise*, **13**, 73–74

Donoghue, S. (1977) The correlation between physical fitness absenteeism and work performance. *Canadian Journal of Public Health*, **68**, 201–203

Fentem, P. H. (1992) Exercise in prevention of disease. *British Medical Bulletin*, **48**, 630–650

Franklin, B. A. (1984) Exercise program compliance. In *Behavioral Management of Obesity* (eds J. Storlie and H. A. Jordan), Human Kinetics, Champaign, Illinois, pp. 106–107

Genaidy, A. M., Bafna, K. M., Sarmidy, R. and Sana, P. (1990) A muscular endurance training program for symmetrical and asymmetrical manual lifting tasks. *Journal of Occupational Medicine* **32**, 226–233

Genaidy, A., Mital, A. and Bafna, K. (1989) An endurance training programme for frequent carrying tasks. *Ergonomics*, **32**, 149–155

Gettman, L. R., Ayres, J. J. and Pollock, M. L. (1978) The effect of circuit weight training on strength, cardio-respiratory function, and body composition of adult men. *Medicine and Science in Sports and Exercise*, **10**, 171–176

Holzbach, R. L., Piserchia, P. V., McFadden, D. W., Hartwell, T. D. Herrmann, A. and Fielding, J. E. (1990) Effect of a comprehensive health promotion program on employee attitudes. *Journal of Occupational Medicine*, **32**, 973–978

Howley, E. T. and Franks, B. D. (1986) *Health/Fitness Instructor's Handbook*, Human Kinetics Publishers, Champaign, Illinois

Janda, V. (1992) *Muscle and Back Pain – Assessment and Treatment of Impaired Movement Patterns and Motor Recruitment*, Associated course to the 5th international symposium of the Physical Medicine Research Foundation (Oxford, 1992)

Kellett, K. M., Kellett, D. A. and Nordholm, L. A. (1991) Effects of an exercise program on sick leave due to back pain. *Physical Therapy*, **71**, 283–293

Lewit, K. (1991) *Manipulative Therapy in Rehabilitation of the Locomotor System*, 2nd edn, Butterworth–Heinemann, Oxford

Lynch, W. D. Golaszewski, T. J., Clearie, A. F., Snow, D. and Vickery, D. M. (1990) Impact of a facility-bases corporate fitness program on the number of absences from work due to illness. *Journal of Occupational Medicine*, **32**, 9–12

McKenzie, R. A. (1981) *The Lumbar Spine. Mechanical Diagnosis and Therapy*, Spinal Pubications, Lower Hutt, New Zealand

Morgan, W. P. (1985) Affective beneficence of vigorous physical activity. *Medicine and Science in Sports and Exercise*, **17**, 94–100

Nachemson, A. (1983) Work for all, for those with low back pain as well. *Clinical Orthopaedics*, **179**, 77–85

Nieman, D. C. and Nehlsen-Cannarella, S. L. (1992) Effects of endurance exercise on the immune response. In *Endurance in Sport* (eds. R. J. Shephard and P.-O. Åstrand), Blackwell Scientific Publications, Oxford, pp. 487–504

Norris, C. M. (1993) *Weight Training. Principles and Practice*, A. and C. Black, London

Pollock, M. L. (1988) Prescribing exercise for fitness and adherence. In: *Exercise Adherence: Its Impact on Public Health* (ed. R. K. Dishman), Human Kinetics Publishers, Champaign, Illinois, 259–277

Renstrom, P. and Kannus, P. (1992) Prevention of injuries in endurance athletes. In *Endurance in Sport* (eds R. J. Shephard and P.-O. Åstrand), Blackwell Scientific Publications, Oxford, pp. 325–350

Richardson, C., Jull, G., Toppenberg, R. and Comerford, M. (1992) Techniques for active lumbar stabilisation for spinal protection: a pilot study. *Australian Journal of Physiotherapy*, **38**, 105–112

Sonstroem, R. J. (1984) Exercise and self esteem. *Exercise and Sports Science Reviews*, **12**, 123–156

Stokes, M. and Young, A. (1984) The contribution of reflex inhibition to arthrogenous muscle weakness. *Clinical Science*, **67**, 7–14

Storlie, J., Baun, W. B. and Horton, W. L. (1992) *Guidelines for Employee Health Promotion Programs. Association for Fitness in Business*, Human Kinetics Publishers, Champaign, Illinois

Tucker, L. A. (1982) Effect of a weight training program on the self concept of college males. *Perceptual and Motor Skills*, **54**, 1055–1061

Vincent, M. F. (1976) Comparison of self-concepts of college women, athletes and physical education majors. *Research Quarterly*, **47**, 218–225

Further reading

American College of Sports Medicine (1986) *Guidelines for Graded Exercise Testing and Exercise Prescription*, 3rd edn, Lea and Febiger, Philadelphia

Ashton, D. and Davies, B. (1986) *Why Exercise?*, Blackwell, Oxford

Fentem, P. H., Bassey, E. J. and Turnbull, N. B. (1988) *The New Case for Exercise*. Health Education Authority, London

Foege, W. H., Bernier, L. L. and Banta, G. R. (1987) Closing the gap: report of the Carter centre health policy consultation. *Journal of the American Medical Association*, **254**, 1416–1421

Norris, C. M. (1993) *Sports Injuries. Diagnosis and Management for Physiotherapist*, Butterworth–Heinemann, Oxford

Patton, R. W., Corry, J. M., Gettman, L. R. and Graf, J. S. (1986) *Implementing Health/Fitness Programs*, Human Kinetics Publishers, Champaign, Illinois

Patton, R. W., Grantham, W. C., Gerson, R. F. and Gettman, L. R. (1989) *Developing and Managing Health/Fitness Facilities*, Human Kinetics Publishers, Champaign, Illinois

Rejeski, W. J. and Kenney, E. A. (1988). *Fitness Motivation. Preventing Participant Dropout*, Life Enhancement Publications, Champagn, Illinois

Chapter 10

Musculoskeletal injury at work: natural history and risk factors

Stephen T. Pheasant

'Work is of two kinds: first, altering the position of matter at or near the earth's surface relatively to other such matter; second, telling other people to do so. The first kind is unpleasant and ill paid; the second is pleasant and highly paid.'

Bertrand Russell (1936) *In Praise of Idleness*

Work can affect your health in a number of ways: sometimes for the better, more often for the worse. The working person may, for example, be exposed to some toxic hazard or similarly injurious chemical, physical or biological agent present in the working environment. Most of the classical 'industrial diseases' are caused in this way – the dust diseases, occupational cancers, dermatitis, noise-induced deafness and so on. Overall, conditions of this sort (with the possible exception of occupational deafness) are becoming rarer, at least in the industrially developed countries, although this is less true of other parts of the world. This tendency is due partly to the better recognition and control of these hazards and partly to changes in the nature of people's work, in that fewer of us are engaged in the sorts of work which expose us to these types of risks. But the classical industrial diseases are in reality just the tip of a very large iceberg of work-related ill health, which may stem from diverse features of the person's working life by processes of injury which are sometimes complex and difficult to pin down precisely.

In many cases the injury which the person sustains (or the condition which he or she develops) stems from the pattern of musculoskeletal loading which the working task entails – as a consequence of the posture in which the task is performed, the required bodily forces and movements, and so on. For the purposes of argument, injuries which are caused in this way are referred to as *ergonomic injuries* and defined thus (Pheasant, 1992a):

> An ergonomic injury is one which results as a direct or indirect consequence of the nature and demands of the person's working task, rather than resulting from some hazard encountered at work which is not intrinsically part of the task itself.

In general, an ergonomic injury results from a *mismatch* between the physical (and sometimes also mental) *demands* of the working task and the *capacity* of the working person to meet those demands (i.e. when the former exceeds the latter).

Ergonomic injuries may occur as discrete events which happen at a particular point in time, either as a result of an *accident* or mischance (see below), or a single episode of *overexertion*. They may occur insidiously over a period of time as the result of *cumulative overuse*. Or, they may result from a combination of both in that the effects of cumulative trauma may render the person susceptible to injury by overexertion. Lifting and handling injuries clearly fall into this category, as do the various work-related upper limb disorders commonly referred to as 'repetitive strain injuries (RSI)'. Insomuch as low back pain is commonly work related, being the result of overexertion or overuse, then back trouble may very often be regarded as an ergonomic injury also. In this chapter, the aetiology of these conditions is discussed in a fairly general way; subsequent chapters will deal with lifting and handling and with RSI in more detail.

Before going any further, however, it is possibly worthwhile pausing to define the word 'injury'. The normal or everyday meaning of the word, as given in the Oxford Dictionary, is: 'harm, damage, wrongful action or treatment'; this is how the author proposes to use the word. There are, however, other indiosyncratic usages – a distinction sometimes being drawn between conditions resulting from acute tissue damage, which are regarded as 'injuries', and other forms of pain and dysfunction, which are not. A certain amount of needless confusion has arisen as a result.

Lifting and handling

According to recent Health and Safety Executive figures (Health and Safety Commission, 1993; Health and Safety Executive, 1993), about one third (32%) of all reported accidents occurring in the workplace are attributable to lifting and handling activities. Of these, a little under half (45%) are injuries to the back; the remainder may affect just about any part of the body. Although these injuries are generally referred to as 'accidents' for administrative purposes, the term is in some respects a little misleading.

An *accident* is an unplanned, unexpected or uncontrolled event – generally one with unhappy consequences. Some manual handling injuries are accidents in this sense of the word, in that some unforeseen mishap occurs which interrupts the normal execution of the lifting action in question. The person may, for example, be injured when a difficult or unstable load gets out of control – because he overbalances and falls, or because he is crushed by the load, or overstrains himself trying to regain control of it. Many manual handling injuries are not accidents in the narrow sense of the word, however, in that there is no intervening unforeseen event other than the direct manifestation of the injury itself – typically a sudden sharp pain in the back, neck, shoulder, wrist, etc. The person is very often performing the lifting action in question in what seems to be an entirely normal way. We could characterize these acute injuries in which there is no specific intervening event as *overexertions*.

Furthermore, in many cases, the action in question is one which the person has performed many times before without suffering any discernible ill effects. What does this tell us? It may be that the individual's physiological capacity for work varies, such that a load which is within his or her safe limit on one occasion is beyond it on another, for example because of acute or chronic fatigue or a virus infection. It is equally possible, however, that some process of cumulative trauma is involved, whereby the individual is rendered progressively susceptible to injury at some point of peak mechanical loading.

It is a matter of common experience that back pain (and other musculoskeletal conditions) may come on following a period of unaccustomedly heavy physical work, whether this be lifting and handling as such or some other biomechanically equivalent activity. Sometimes, these episodes are transient and we regard them as everyday postexercise muscle soreness. In other cases, the resolution of the condition is delayed and we regard them as 'injuries' of a more severe kind. The period of exposure to the activity in question may be one of hours or days, but in either case one must suppose that the mechanism of injury is one of cumulative trauma or overuse of the tissues concerned.

Given that heavy physical work may result in a process of cumulative injury in the medium/short term, it stands to reason that it may be similarly injurious over a longer time scale. There is good epidemiological evidence that this is the case. It has been known for many years that people in heavy jobs will (at any given age) show more advanced signs of osteoarthritic degeneration of the lumbar spine (but not the cervical spine) than people in lighter jobs (Hult, 1955). More recently, Kumar (1990) found a statistical association between back pain and the cumulative biomechanical loading to which the person's spine had been exposed during the course of his or her working life.

To summarize, therefore, lifting and handling tasks entail risks of:

- accidental injury
- overexertion
- cumulative overuse.

Repetitive strain injury

The term repetitive strain injury as it is customarily used, refers to a generic category of overuse injuries affecting the forearm, wrist and hand and (perhaps to a lesser extent) the neck and shoulder region and proximal parts of the upper limb. These conditions occur in people doing a variety of kinds of repetitive or otherwise hand-intensive work, particularly industrial assembly line workers and keyboard users, but also agricultural and craft workers, musicians, and so on.

The term RSI has been widely deprecated, there being those who argue that RSI is not caused by repetition, that it is not a strain and not an injury. The first two points are, in the author's view, well made. Repetitive motions are but one of a number of causative factors leading to the onset of these conditions (static muscle loading is probably equally important if not more so), and the conditions which fall into the RSI generic category are not in most cases 'strains' in the normal medical sense of the word. The assertion that RSI is not an injury is, at the end of the day, solely a matter of semantics and just what one takes the word 'injury' to mean. A certain amount of sterile and somewhat tedious debate has revolved around this point. It seems perfectly clear to the author that the people with RSI whom he sees on a day-to-day basis, are injured in every normal sense of the word (see definition above).

The term RSI originated in Australia and has been widely taken up in the UK, at least by the general public. In North America, a broadly similar range of conditions are referred to as cumulative trauma disorders, and in some other countries they are known as occupational cervicobrachial disorders (OCD). In Australasia, the controversy surrounding RSI in the popular media has led to the term being abandoned in favour of occupational overuse syndrome (OOS); and in the UK the officially condoned term is work-related upper limb disorders (WRULD). It must be emphasized that all these terms mean much the same thing; and all are inexact in that they refer to a class of conditions rather than a single clinical entity.

The use of generic terms of this kind has certain advantages, particularly in the medicolegal context, in that it enables us to place an injury within a class of conditions which are held to result from common causative factors, without necessarily having to reach a precise clinical diagnosis in any particular case. The principal occupational or ergonomic risk factors leading to the onset of these conditions are summarized in Table 10.1.

The use of generic terms of this kind also has disadvantages, however. The first is that they make too strong a distinction between overuse injuries to the neck, shoulder and upper limb and conditions of similar aetiology affecting other parts of the body. The distinction is justified up to a point. Cervical spine dysfunction and other conditions leading to nerve entrapment at the thoracic outlet or more distally may lead to pain radiating down the limb; likewise, trigger points in proximal muscle groups may refer pain to more distal sites. There is also a marked propensity for the symptoms of these conditions to 'spread' – from proximal to

Table 10.1 Ergonomic risk factors

Repetitive strain injury
Frequent or repeated gripping and turning actions
Force exertion
Wrist deviation
Static muscle loading (often postural)
Prolonged intensive keyboard use
Lack of task diversity
Unaccustomed physical activity
Vibration
Psychological factors

Back pain
Heavy work: lifting, pushing, pulling, sudden maximal force
    exertion, bending, twisting, etc.
Stooped working posture
Prolonged sedentary work
Lack of task diversity
Unaccustomed physical activity
Vibration
Psychosocial factors

distal or vice versa (see below). Furthermore, it is not uncommon for jobs which involve frequent hand and wrist movements to involve a static loading on neck and shoulder muscles also, entailing a risk of overuse injury at both proximal and distal sites; this is true of both keyboard work and the repetitive hand-intensive tasks of the industrial assembly line.

On the basis of these considerations, therefore, it is entirely reasonable to regard occupational overuse injuries to the neck, shoulder and upper limb as constituting a meaningful class or category. Occupational overuse injuries to the upper limb have received a considerable degree of attention, both in the scientific literature and the popular media. But they are by no means unique. A similar class of conditions affecting the lower limb has been described (Marr, 1985) and, as will be argued in due course, the similarities between these disorders and work-related conditions affecting the lumbar spine and other axial musculoskeletal structures are probably greater than the differences.

The second disadvantages of the RSI/OOS/WRULD generic label is the diversity of conditions to which it is applied. Some of these are relatively discrete and localized clinical entities which are relatively uncontentious, in that there is a broad measure of agreement concerning their underlying pathology and the diagnostic signs and symptoms by which they may be recognized. Conditions of this sort include: the various forms of tenosynovitis and peritendinitis affecting the tendons of the forearm flexors and extensors; lateral and medial epicondylitis; carpal tunnel syndrome, and so on. These are sometimes referred to as type I RSI (Littlejohn and Miller, 1986).

In very many cases, however (perhaps as many as 90%), no such precise diagnosis is possible, in that the patient does not present with any sufficiently clear pattern of signs and symptoms such as would enable him (or more commonly her) to be allocated to any specific clinical category of known underlying pathology. These latter cases are sometimes referred to as type II RSI; in a recent paper on the subject, these were referred to as RSI of unknown pathology or RSI(UP) – although in retrospect it would be better to characterize their underlying pathology as obscure or disputed rather than unknown (Pheasant, 1992b). Conditions of this more obscure sort occur particularly commonly in intensive keyboard users – data processing workers, copy typists, legal secretaries, and so on – although they are by no means unknown in hand-intensive blue collar jobs. They are characterized by diffuse pain and dysfunction, with palpable tenderness at multiple sites, most commonly the 1st dorsal interosseous, the muscle bellies of the forearm flexors and extensors, the medial and lateral epicondyles, the upper arm in the vicinity of the bicipital groove, the upper trapezius and rhomboids, and in some cases the quadratus lumborum and even in lower limb muscle groups. In addition there will be very often (but not invariably) signs of 'adverse mechanical tension' affecting the roots or branches of the brachial plexus, as evidence by a positive upper limb tension test (see, for example, Butler, 1991). Some patients also show signs of vasomotor disturbance, which in advanced cases may be sufficiently severe to warrant being described as a reflex sympathetic dystrophy. This is thought to be a complication of the basic condition resulting from disuse of the affected limb. To make matters more complicated, it is by no means uncommon for a patient to suffer from both the localized (type I) and diffuse (type II) forms of RSI – either at the same time or at different stages in the history of the condition – and it is worth noting that when this is the case, direct medical or surgical treatments aimed at the alleviation of the localized condition tend to be of relatively limited success in dealing with the syndrome as a whole.

The natural history of the diffuse forms of RSI is variable: onset may be rapid or gradual; development of the condition is very often progressive. The first symptom is commonly a localized tingling in the hands or aching at the wrist, which comes on at work and is relieved by rest. In typists, it is commonly the left hand that is affected first, notwithstanding that he/she may be right/handed, and indeed the left side will often be affected more severely at all stages. The person concerned often finds this puzzling, but it is not really so surprising when one considers that in typing ordinary English text on a conventional 'QWERTYUIOP' keyboard, the fingers of the left hand make around 30% more keystrokes than the right. In data entry workers, who mainly use the numerical keypad, the right hand is usually affected first and more severely. In some cases it is possible to attribute specific patterns of symptoms (affecting individual fingers) to idiosyncratic patterns of keyboard use.

These initially localized symptoms may become progressively more severe over a period of several months, the progression often being accelerated at a time of unusually heavy workload. The pain comes on earlier in the working day and begins to affect non-occupational 'mundane' uses of the hand. At about the same time, symptoms begin to 'spread', from distal to proximal or proximal to distal as the case may be (more commonly the former). Symptoms which were initially unilateral may come to affect the contralateral upper limb, and in some cases may even spread down the back and even to lower limbs sites. This spreading may in part be due to altered body mechanics – the person may 'favour' the injured limb in the performance of everyday activities and thus initiate an overuse injury to the opposite limb – but it is probably much more a consequence of the underlying pathology of the condition.

The pathophysiology of diffuse or type II RSI is contentious. Setting aside the views of people who misguidedly regard this condition as 'all in the mind' or the product of hysteria (Lucire, 1986), there are two principal views worthy of consideration at the present time. The first regards the condition as essentially myalgic, in that it is in part due to an overuse injury to muscle or myofascial tissue and in part the results of neurological sensitization (i.e. physiological changes in the CNS mechanism which mediate the experience of pain), which in turn may have a psychological component, particularly in the chronic stages. This is essentially the position the author adopted in an earlier book (Pheasant, 1991) and it has been stated subsequently in greater detail by Cohen et al. (1992). A recent publication of the New Zealand Occupational Safety and Health Service (OSH, 1992) takes up much the same position, and the views of Huskisson (1992) are not altogether dissimilar, although to my mind he places undue emphasis on the psychogenic component of the disorder. (He also, slightly unconventionally, restricts the term RSI to the diffuse forms.)

A fair amount of experimental evidence has emerged in support of the position described above. Dennett and Fry (1988) took biopsy specimens from the hand muscles of RSI sufferers and normal volunteers. The muscle tissue from the RSI sufferers showed a number of abnormalities at the microscopic level, which would be reasonable to regard as signs of physical damage. Differences between patients and controls were statistically significant, and the extent of these signs of damage was roughly proportional to the severity of the individual's clinical symptoms. The findings of Dennet and Fry have subsequently been confirmed by Lindman et al. (1991), who found broadly similar histological abnormalities in biopsy specimens taken from the upper trapezius muscles of Swedish assembly line workers. The neurological element has also been demonstrated experimentally – by Helme et al. (1992) who found physiological evidence of altered nociceptive function in RSI patients. Findings of this sort are important not only in that they provide us with a starting point for understanding the underlying pathology of the diffuse forms of RSI, but also because they provide clear and incontrovertible evidence that these conditions have a foundation in organic pathology and are therefore by no means 'all in the mind', as some people still like to claim.

The second principal view on the subject, sometimes called the 'neurogenic hypothesis of RSI', – is that the diffuse forms are principally the consequence of nerve entrapment (see Butler, 1991; Quintner and Elvey, 1991).

The principal strength of the latter view is that clinical experience is increasingly indicating that methods of treatment based on this theory tend to be more effective than other therapeutic approaches to the problem. The principal strength of the former view, in addition to the mounting body of experimental evidence in its support, is that it explains most of the observables of the aetiology and natural history of the condition. Doubtless these two viewpoints will be reconciled in due course and such new theories as emerge will encompass elements of both.

It is increasingly clear, however, that notwithstanding the

diversity of natural history of these conditions and the disputed status of their underlying pathology, the diffuse forms of RSI are sufficiently consistent in their clinical manifestations to be regarded as a specific clinical entity in their own right, independently of the localized conditions like tenosynovitis. For better or for worse – and more by default than otherwise – this entity is coming to be known as the *repetitive strain syndrome*. (It is recognized that the term is in many ways an unfortunate one but there would be little to be gained at the present time by inventing yet another alternative.)

The natural history of the work-related upper limb disorders is, however, more complex still. Conditions like de Quervain's tenosynovitis, especially as they occur in blue collar workers, typically have a relatively acute onset, which is very often associated with a change in working practices, period of unaccustomed work or abnormally heavy workload (which imposes an unusual pattern of biomechanical loading), or with the return to work after a period of absence (during which time the person may be presumed to have become 'deconditioned' to the activity in question). Indeed, it is by no means unknown for tenosynovitis to arise as the result of an acute overexertion injury. With rest and conservative management, acute tenosynovitis generally resolves in a matter of a few weeks or a month or two at the most. But in a minority of cases a chronic condition of a more obscure sort may supervene, the definitive signs of tenosynovitis *per se* being no longer present. Cases of this sort become particularly contentious in the medicolegal context. They are, in the author's view, best regarded as a *post-tenosynovitis syndrome* which stems from the initial injury. The extent to which this condition is the same as the *repetitive strain syndrome* described above is at present unclear.

Back pain at work

Back pain is a major problem throughout the developed world (and in all likelihood elsewhere, had we the data to know). In 1990 some 60 million working days were lost to

British industry as a result of back pain. The economic cost of this sickness absence has been placed at some £3 billion – or about the equivalent of the combined annual turnover of GEC, Ferranti and Kodak (National Back Pain Association, 1991). In New Zealand, where all accidental injuries are by law compensatable (however caused), back injuries account for about a quarter of all monies thus paid out. What is worse, back pain sickness absence is increasing rapidly on an upwardly accelerating curve and, curiously enough, is increasing more rapidly in women than in men (Pheasant 1992a).

It has been known for very many years that people who do heavy manual work are more likely to suffer with their backs than people in lighter occupations. In statistical terms, however, the difference is perhaps surprisingly small, except when it comes to long-term disability and sickness absence (Hult, 1955; Pheasant, 1991). Basically, this is because the relationship between back pain prevalence and physical workload is U-shaped: people in physically very demanding jobs are at risk, as are people whose work is fully sedentary; but people whose jobs involve moderate physical demands fall into a low-risk category, particularly if these jobs also have postural diversity (i.e. the person spends part of the time sitting and part standing). This is clear from the classic epidemiological studies of Magora (1972), and has recently been confirmed in cadaveric studies by Videman et al. (1990). On the basis of Magora's prevalence figures, it has been argued that the magnitude of the difference between occupational categories (approximately 10:1) is such that some 85% of all episodes of back pain occurring in the working population may be regarded as work related – in other words they may be regarded as ergonomic injuries (Pheasant, 1991). Occupational or ergonomic risk factors for low back pain are summarized in Table 10.1.

About half of all episodes of back pain are acute in their onset and in about half of cases the onset is insidious, with the person in question very often being at a loss to attribute the episode to any particular cause; see Figure 10.1. There is some evidence to suggest that first attacks are more likely to be insidious and recurrences acute, but this has not been

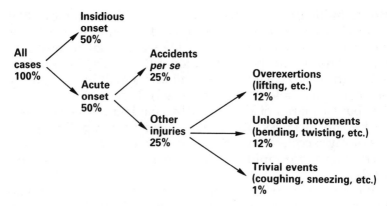

Fig. 10.1 Onset of back pain.

explored in much detail (Peter Buckle, 1993, personal communication). Of the episodes of acute onset, about half are the result of accidents as such (in the meaning of the word defined above). Of the remainder, about half can be classed as overexertion injuries, in that the person is engaged in some strenuous physical activity (like lifting, etc.) at the time in question. However, about half are associated with bodily movements such as bending or twisting where no great degree of exertion is involved, and a small minority are associated with seemingly trivial things like coughing or sneezing, etc. The inference to be drawn is that the levels of biomechanical loading required to cause an acute back injury are variable in the extreme – which implies that some people are very much more vulnerable to injury than others. The reasons for this vulnerability are in all probability manifold; prior injury from which recovery has been incomplete and the effects of cumulative trauma are probably an important part of the picture in many cases. This has important implications when it comes to setting load limits for lifting and handling (see Pheasant, 1991 for a detailed discussion of this problem).

A detailed appraisal of those personal characteristics which place an individual at risk is beyond the scope of the present text. A previous history of back trouble is the most important. After that come things like a low degree of overall fitness, physical strength which is not up to the demands of the task, cigarette smoking and motherhood. (Risk of serious back injury increases with number of children for women but not for men, probably partly because of the stresses to the spine which results from pregnancy and childbirth and partly because of the physical workload entailed in looking after young children.) The predictive value of factors other than these is relatively poor. This analysis has important implications when it comes to selecting and screening people for heavy occupations (Pheasant, 1991).

Back pain and RSI

It is all to easy to regard back injury and RSI as two separate issues. In reality, the similarities are probably very much greater than the differences. A precise clinical diagnosis pointing to a condition of known underlying pathology is probably possible in only 10–20% of cases of back pain (Kersley, 1979; Pheasant, 1991). The same could be said for RSI. It is probable, furthermore, that in the majority of cases (of both back pain and RSI) where no such precise diagnosis is possible, the underlying condition is essentially myalgic (see above), with elements of nerve entrapment and/or joint dysfunction being involved at least in some cases. The symptoms of RSI may spread from distal to proximal or vice versa, and in some cases may come to affect the muscles of the trunk and lower limbs. It has likewise been shown that people who suffer from low back pain are statistically more likely to suffer from neck pain also and vice versa (Hult, 1955; Pheasant, 1991). As with the 'spreading' of RSI, this may in part be the result of altered body mechanics and in part a consequence of the underlying neurophysiology of the condition.

Consider the lists of risk factors in Table 10.1; they are really remarkably similar. By comparison with back pain and RSI, occupational overuse injuries to the lower limbs have not received much attention – perhaps because people just soldier on when their feet hurt. But there seems little reason to imagine that were the appropriate studies to be performed the risk factors would turn out to be very different, although doubtless there would be additional ones like poorly-fitting shoes and hard flooring materials.

Both back pain and RSI are conditions of diverse natural history in terms of their onset and their outcome. It is to the latter exceedingly important issue that we shall now turn.

Recurrence and chronicity

Most episodes of back pain are relatively short, with the symptoms clearing up in a week or two at the most. The problem is that back trouble tends to be recurrent and in a minority of cases becomes chronic. Around 50% of people recovering from an acute episode of back trouble will have another episode during the following year, and the probability of a recurrence increases with the number of previous attacks. There seem to be two principal patterns of recurrence. Some people (who are often middle aged or older) have periodic attacks, but in their pain-free intervals are capable of relatively demanding physical work. Others (who may be any age) are never really pain free. They typically describe themselves as suffering from a dull ache (which is not necessarily very well localized) more or less all of the time, which periodically flares up into episodes of intense pain (although not necessarily always in the same part of the back). The ongoing dull ache is commonly made worse by specific activities (prolonged stooping, standing, sitting, etc.), which in the worse cases may precipitate the acute flare-ups (Troup et al., 1981; Pheasant, 1991). These two patterns of recurrence could be characterized as *episodic* and *acute on chronic*, respectively.

Although most periods of back pain sickness absence are relatively short, the distribution is skewed, with a minority of cases leading to long-term disability. About 5% of episodes lead to a period off work lasting 3 months or more. There is evidence that this minority of chronic cases accounts for a disproportionately large slice of the economic loss associated with back pain (about 85% according to some sources); and although these things are very much more difficult to quantify it seems likely that this must also be true for the human costs of back pain in terms of pain and suffering, loss of amenity, quality of life, and so on. It has been estimated that after 6 months' absence an individual's chance of ever returning to work has fallen to about 50%; after 1 year to 25%; and after 2 years to virtually nil. Back care programmes and other measures aimed at the prevention of back pain in the workplace must therefore be planned at two levels:

1. Primary: prevention of injury
2. Secondary: prevention of recurrence and progression to chronicity.

The factors which underlie the progression to chronicity are contentious. The two principal conflicting viewpoints in this area may be summed up in the following propositions:

Proposition 1. Back pain is commonly work related. If you fix a person up after an acute episode and send him back to work without eliminating the features of his working life which caused the problem in the first place, then it will be scarcely surprising if his condition recurs or becomes chronic. The progression to chronicity results for re-injury of the anatomical structures in question, and a progressively increasing susceptibility to injury due to cumulative damage to these structures.

Proposition 2. Chronic back pain is not an injury at all; it is rather the result of a downward spiral of inactivity and diminished functional capacity, which is contingent upon inappropriate pain avoidance behaviour, a depressed mood state and the adoption of 'the sick role'. The best way to prevent this cycle from becoming established is to encourage the earliest possible return to a full range of everyday activities, including work.

The author has argued strongly for the first of these propositions in an earlier book (Pheasant, 1991). We have no real reason to regard these propositions as mutually exclusive however – at least not in any absolute sense – although this may appear to be the case insomuch as the two positions are often adopted for adversarial purposes in the medicolegal context. Both propositions are reductionist: the former sees the problem solely in physical terms; the latter solely in psychosocial terms. Both are therefore incomplete. Furthermore, there is little doubt that chronic pain is fundamentally different from acute pain, both physiologically in terms of the underlying neural mechanisms involved, and psychologically in terms of its meaning for the individual concerned.

The apparent contradiction between these viewpoints can be resolved if chronic back pain is regarded as a *post-injury syndrome*, the development of which involves elements of:

- physical re-injury
- neurological sensitization
- changes contingent on disuse
- psychosocial reinforcement.

The concept of the post-injury syndrome (as noted above with regard to tenosynovitis) is as relevant to RSI and other work-related musculoskeletal injuries as it is to chronic back trouble. The concept has important medicolegal consequences in that the direct cause of the initial injury – whether this be an acute event, cumulative trauma or a mixture of both – may be regarded as the cause at law of the final chronic state, given that the *chain of causation* remains unbroken by any identifiable external intervening event.

At this point it is appropriate to attempt to summarize the natural history of musculoskeletal injury at work in terms of both the mode of onset and the outcome. The principal possibilities are set out in Table 10.2. The aetiology of these conditions is summarized in block diagram form in Figure 10.2. It must be emphasized that this is only a summary; there are doubtless numerous other pathways and feedback loops in the system. The reader might care to try to think of some of these and draw his/her own block diagram.

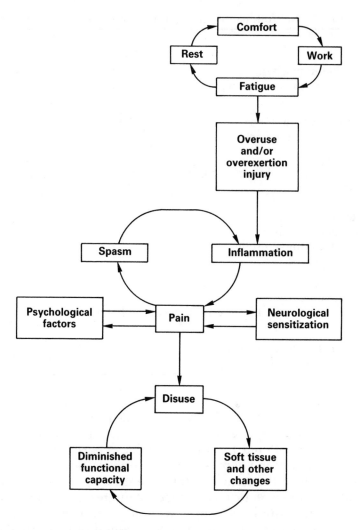

Fig. 10.2 Ergonomic injury and the post-injury syndrome.

Psychological aspects

All pain and disability has a psychological dimension; to deny this is to regard the person as a mere mechanism. The pain

Table 10.2 Natural history of ergonomic injuries

Onset
Acute
  Accident/mischance
  Overexertion (no intervening event)

Subacute
  Onset over hours or days, often as a result of some
    unaccustomed activity

Insidious
  Onset over weeks months or years, as a result of cumulative
    trauma

Outcome
Transient episode
  Resolves uneventfully

Recurrent
  Episodic
  Acute on chronic
  Episodes may be triggered by specific activities

Chronic
  Progressive/degenerative
  Postinjury syndrome

and disability which results from musculoskeletal injury is no exception. Frymoyer et al. (1980), for example, found that people who suffered from back trouble reported more episodes of anxiety and depression than controls; Bowden (1991) reported much the same for RSI sufferers.

Vallfors (1985) reported a number of interesting findings in a comparative study of people with acute and chronic back trouble, the latter being defined by a period of more than 3 months' sickness absence. On careful clinical examination, Vallfors was unable to demonstrate objective physical signs in 70% of chronic cases as against 40% of acute cases (One might perhaps expect this from the subsidence of acute inflammation, etc.). The chronic cases were also a psychologically distinguishable group, showing more signs of psychological illness and alcohol abuse and reporting lower levels of job satisfaction. Of these chronic cases some 31% believed, however, that it was their working conditions which prevented them from returning to work. There was a certain amount of evidence that this perception of the matter was a valid one, in that conversations with their foremen confirmed that their working conditions were in many cases bad or very bad. It may well be, therefore, that their low levels of reported job satisfaction were (in part at least) attributable to the fact that they had unsatisfactory jobs.

More recently, in a now widely celebrated prospective study of employees in the Boeing organization, Bigos et al. (1991) found that a low degree of job satisfaction and certain personality traits were better predictors of reported back injury than things like lifting strengths, cardiorespiratory fitness, spinal flexibility and task demands (as assessed by a computerized technique of biomechanical analysis). Before jumping to too strong a conclusion on the basis of this study, it should be noted that a previous history of back trouble was also a very strong predictor; it may be that the psychosocial factors noted here are in fact markers of the progression to chronicity rather than the initial process of injury itself (or the reporting of that injury, as the authors suggest). In addition, the absence of an association with task demands may well be a consequence of the particular method of biomechanical analysis which was used and the U-shaped risk curve (see above). Having said this, occupational psychologists have recognized for many years that sickness absence (and by analogy the reporting of injury) is in part determined by psychosocial factors.

In a case control study of data entry workers with and without symptoms of RSI, Ryan and Bampton (1988) found something rather similar. Cases had palpable tender points at multiple sites (as described above), and reported more stress and boredom at work and lower degrees of autonomy, peer group cohesion and role clarity. There is evidence, however, that these psychologically adverse appraisals of the working situation are, in part at least, the reflection of objective features of the individual's working life, rather than some personal idiosyncrasy of the individual worker. In a comparison of organizations doing similar sorts of keyboard work but having high and low prevalences of RSI, Hopkins (1990) used the questionnaire responses of symptom-free workers only. Those in the high prevalence workplaces reported higher degrees of stress and boredom, and lower degrees of autonomy, task variety, peer group cohesion and job satisfaction. In other words, those features of working life which distinguished sufferers from non-sufferers in the former study also distinguished non-sufferers in high prevalence organizations from those in low prevalence organizations in the latter study, suggesting that the problem lies (at least in part) with the organization rather than the individual.

To some extent, associations of this kind may be explained by the fact that many of the features of working life which make a job stressful, boring and psychologically distasteful – excessive workload, repetitiveness, lack of task diversity and so on – are also likely to be physically injurious. But it is probably more complex than this. Back pain and RSI are conditions of complex and multifactorial aetiology in which both physical and psychosocial risk factors may play a part, and the latter perhaps become increasingly dominant as these conditions progress to their chronic forms.

It is, at least in principle, possible to propose a number of possible theories to account for the observed association between chronic musculoskeletal conditions like back pain and RSI and the states of anxiety and depression which the people who suffer these injuries so commonly experience. Five possibilities are summarized in Table 10.3. In the author's view the probability is that all of these theories (other than theory 3) contain some elements of truth, and their validity and explanatory values may well vary from case to case.

It is unfortunately all too easy to allow the distinction between the psychosocial component of chronic musculoskeletal injury and outright malingering to become blurred. The distinction is a vital one. Malingering is an act of conscious deceit. Malingering as such – although not unknown – is, in the view of all informed people, relatively rare. The work-injured person who is trapped in a downward spiral of disablement and despair (which can lead in the most severe cases to suicide) is not in any sense whatsoever a malingerer.

Table 10.3 Psychological factors in chronic musculoskeletal pain

Theory 1

Chronic musculoskeletal pain and dysfunction are (sometimes) caused by work. The same features of work which cause musculoskeletal injury may be psychologically stressful. This stress may become manifest in changes of mood state – anxiety, depression, etc.

Theory 2

Chronic pain and disability are of themselves depressing and are a legitimate source of anxiety

Theory 3

Chronic pain and disability are (sometimes) the outward and visible manifestations of an inner psychological state of disturbance or distress. Symptoms which superficially appear to be musculoskeletal may in fact be the product of somatization or hysterical conversion. This externalization of the person's inner conflicts may provide both primary and secondary gain for the individual concerned

Theory 4

Chronic pain and disability are the result of a downward spiral of inactivity and diminished functional capacity contingent upon inappropriate pain avoidance behaviour and the adopting of 'the sick role'. This cycle is more likely to become established in a person who is depressed; such a person will find it more difficult to break out of this spiral once it has become established

Theory 5

Chronic musculoskeletal pain, depression and lethargy may all be manifestations of the same neurochemical dysfunction or imbalance; non-restorative sleep may be part of the same picture, possibly as an intervening variable

Theory 5a

People who suffer from this neurochemical imbalance (perhaps as a result of some hereditary predisposition) may be more vulnerable to injury in high-risk working situations, or may be more likely to develop a chronic condition following a relatively trivial injury

The imputation of malingering which so commonly arises is both inhumane and deeply offensive to the truly work-injured person; to accuse the despairing victim of chronic back trouble or RSI of being a malingerer is wholly wrong.

Summary and conclusions

This chapter has provided arguments in favour of the concepts of an ergonomic injury and the post-injury syndrome. Furthermore, it has been argued that the similarities between back trouble and the class of conditions called RSI or work-related upper limb disorders are greater than the differences, both conditions being principally the consequence of occupational overuse, notwithstanding their complex multifactorial aetiology in which both physical and psychosocial risk factors may play a part (the latter being increasingly important as the condition progresses to its chronic stages).

The challenge is to develop effective strategies for both primary and secondary prevention, the former being based upon an adequate recognition of the diversity of the risk factors involved and the latter on an adequate recognition of the complexity of the processes which lead to chronicity. The consequence of failing to do so is the appalling waste of human potential which these conditions currently entail.

References

Bigos, S.J., Battie, P.T., Spengler, D.M. et al. (1991) A prospective study of work perceptions and psychosocial factors affecting the report of back injury. *Spine*, **16**, 1–6

Bowden, L. (1991) *Precipitating Factors and Psychological Consequences of Repetition Strain Injury and Personality Characteristics of Sufferers*, unpublished dissertation, Royal Holloway and New College, University of London

Butler, D.S. (1991) *Mobilization of the Nervous System*, Churchill Livingstone, London

Cohen, M.L., Arroyo, J.F., Champion, G.D. and Browne, D. (1992)

In search of the pathogenesis of refractory cervicobrachial pain syndrome. A reconstruction of the RSI phenomenon. *Medical Journal of Australia*, **156**, 432–436

Dennet, X. and Fry, H.J.H. (1988) Overuse syndrome: a muscle biopsy study. *Lancet*, **i**, 905–908

Frymoyer, J.W., Pope, M.H., Constanza, M.C., Rosen, J.C., Coggin, J.E. and Wilder, D.G. (1980) Epidemiological studies of low-back pain. *Spine*, **5**, 419–423

Health and Safety Commission (1993) *Annual Report 1992/93*. HSE Books, London

Health and Safety Executive (1993) *Manual Handling Guidance Regulations*. HMSO, London

Helme, R.D., LeVasseur, S.A. and Gibson, S.J. (1992) RSI revisited: evidence for psychological and physiological differences from an age, sex and occupation matched control group. *Australia and New Zealand Medical Journal*, **22**, 23–29

Hopkins, A. (1990) Stress, the quality of work and repetition strain injury in Australia. *Work and Stress*, **4**, 129–138

Hult, L. (1955) Cervical, dorsal and lumbar spine syndromes. *Acta Orthopaedica Scandinavica*, Suppl. 17

Huskisson, E. (1992) *Repetitive Strain Injury. The Keyboard Disease*, Charterhouse, London

Kersley, G.D. (1979) Back pain: its problems and treatment. *Current Medical Research and Opinion*, **6** (Suppl. 2), 27–32

Kumar, S. (1990) Cumulative load as a risk factor for back pain. *Spine*, **15**, 1311–1316

Lindman, R., Hagberg, M., Angqvist, K.-A., Soderlund, K., Hultman, E. and Thornell, L.-E. (1991) Changes in muscle morphology in chronic trapezius myalgia. *Scandinavian Journal of Work Environment and Health*, **17**, 347–355

Littlejohn, G.O. and Miller, M.H. (1986) Repetitive strain injury: divide and conquer. *Australian Family Physician*, **15**, 409–413

Lucire, Y. (1986) Neurosis in the workplace. *Medical Journal of Australia*, **145**, 323–330

Magor, A. (1972) Investigations of the relation between low back pain and occupation III. Physical requirements: sitting, standing and weight lifting. *Industrial Medicine*, **41**, 5–9

Marr, S.J. (1985) Overuse syndrome of the lower limbs. *Journal of Occupational Health and Safety of Australia and New Zealand*, **1**, 130–134

National Back Pain Association (1991) *Annual Report 1990–1991*. NBPA, Teddington, Middlesex

Occupational Safety and Health Service (1992) *Occupational Overuse*

Syndrome. Treatment and Rehabilitation: A Practitioner's Guide, OSH, Department of Labour, Wellington, New Zealand

Pheasant, S.T. (1991) *Ergonomics, Work and Health*, Macmillan, London

Pheasant, S.T. (1992a) Ergonomics – the design of work. *Impact of Science on Society*, **165**, 3–12

Pheasant, S.T. (1992b) Does RSI exist? *Occupational Medicine*, **42**, 167–168

Quintner, J. and Elvey, R. (1991) *The Neurogenic Hypothesis of RSI*, Working Paper No. 24, National Centre for Epidemiology and Population Health, The Australian National University, Canberra

Ryan, G.A. and Bampton, M. (1988) Comparison of data processing operators with and without upper limb symptoms. *Community Health Studies*, **12**, 63–68

Troup, J.D.G., Martin, J.W. and Lloyd, D.C.E. (1981) Back pain in industry: a prospective study. *Spine*, **6**, 61–69

Vallfors, B. (1985) Acute, subacute, and chronic low back pain – clinical symptoms, absenteeism and working environment. *Scandinavian Journal of Rehabilitation Medicine*, Suppl. 11, 1–98

Videman, T., Nurminen, M. and Troup, J.D.G. (1990) Lumbar spinal pathology in cadaveric material in relation to history of low back pain, occupation and physical loading. *Spine*, **8**, 728–740

Chapter 11

Moving and handling

Joan C. Gabbett
Gillian M. Oldham

Moving and handling of loads together with tripping, slipping and falling have always been recognized as a major cause of work-related accidents with their associated sickness, disability and loss of productivity. All cause damage to the musculoskeletal system and are often linked in actual situations, such as slipping whilst carrying a load. However, it is a fallacy to believe that every injury to the musculoskeletal system is caused by an accident. It may be that the employee relates the pain and discomfort felt to a single incident or accident, but injuries can originate days, weeks, months or even years earlier when the body was first regularly subjected to the stress and strain of microtrauma. Initially this goes unnoticed, but over time cumulatively adds up and reaches a point where discomfort and pain is felt (McKenzie, 1983).

The Health and Safety Executive estimated that the total annual cost to the country of musculoskeletal disease among the working population exceeded £25 billion (Health and Safety Commission, 1991). Handling injuries often involve long periods of sickness absence, which is costly for the employer and the employee in both financial and human terms. The employer must bear the cost of sickness absence and all its associated administrative costs which can include the cost of recruiting, training and supervising a replacement. If the injured employee does return to work, his/her efficiency may be permanently impaired and rehabilitation or job relocation may be necessary. Any accident or injury renders the employer liable to legal action. Claims are costly and the numbers are rising. The landmark case in the NHS is that of Williams *v* Gwent health authority in 1982 where the health authority was held liable for having an unsafe system of work (National Back Pain Association and Royal College of Nursing, 1992). Since that breakthrough nurses have become increasingly litigious. For any organization the costs of legal action are daunting and must be added to any compensation awarded which can be for pain and suffering, as well as loss of career and future loss of earnings.

The employees in turn face a threat to job, income and lifestyle due to residual disability and pain. Fear and memory of pain can reduce confidence in their ability to do the job and work normally and they may worry about the increased risk of further injury or other problems. Fear and anxiety can in themselves increase pain and disability. The work still has to be done, often resulting in colleagues shouldering the work of the injured employee in addition to their own, further widening mental and physical stress. The way that an employer treats an injured employee can have a considerable effect on the morale of co-employees. Therapists, injured workers and employers often seem less positive and optimistic about return of function after back injury than after other musculoskeletal injuries or illness. Good early treatment and advice and regular monitoring, with a phased return to normal working time and intensity, all of which are within the role of the occupational health (OH) physiotherapist, should help to overcome this prejudice and prove that good recovery is possible after back injury.

Early attempts to reduce the costs and human suffering of work-related injuries were directed primarily towards the prevention of accidents. When this approach failed to halt the escalating amount of sickness absence due to musculoskeletal illness, it became more widely accepted that emphasis must be placed on the avoidance and prevention of cumulative stress and strain. This has been reflected in recent legislation and regulations, as well as in the preventive measures being used by occupational health workers.

Physiotherapists have many skills to bring to the moving and handling team. They can make rapid visual assessments of posture and movement and foresee the effects of changing working heights or postures. Their knowledge of human biomechanics, physiology, anthropometry and analysis of posture seem to be rare skills outside the sporting world. They have detailed understanding of how 'normal' bodies are affected by a range of changes, from those of ageing to the effects of generalized illness or specific localized problems of the human locomotor system, and how each affects the performance of manual tasks including moving and handling. Physiotherapists are also aware of the wide range of 'normal' that exists whether one talks about body type, joint mobility, strength, co-ordination or mental attitude. An understanding of how fatigue, boredom, stress and anxiety affect movement is crucial in unravelling why some moving and handling tasks go wrong and cause injury. It is failure to take into account all these human variables which can render policies for, and training in, moving and handling ineffective.

The routine work of OH departments in monitoring the health of employees and trying to ensure their long-term well-being is an important issue in moving and handling. At pre-employment medicals, the physiotherapist can assess potential employees who are found to have pre-existing musculoskeletal conditions which could affect their manual handling abilities. Regular monitoring of employees who have chronic health problems or who are returning to work following sickness absence is invaluable. An individual's ability to perform manual tasks can be compromised by a wide range of medical conditions which do not necessarily involve the musculoskeletal system directly, and may not in any way be caused by work, but which may be aggravated by it.

The OH physiotherapist can assess functional ability and advise management on safe working limits for individual employees (as well as groups). The likelihood of further sickness absence or injury can be much reduced by careful supervision and the use of work restrictions. It is ideal if staff can either return part-time or to light duties, gradually increasing working time and duties as they gain confidence in their ability to cope, until they are working as normally as possible. In other countries, and to some extent in the UK, various strengthening, flexibility and work hardening exercises are being evaluated in an effort to increase efficiency of new and existing workers and reduce lost time (Genaidy et al., 1992). Some organizations also provide gymnasiums and other sporting facilities for staff, that can be used not only to increase overall fitness but also as part of a rehabilitation or prevention scheme.

Sociological and demographic issues

No attempt can be made to prevent injury and strain without some understanding of changes in characteristics of the working population and background of working practice.

The proportion of workers engaged in manufacturing industry in the UK has fallen year on year and been matched by a progressive increase in clerical and office workers (*Employment Gazette*, 1993). The balance is made up by the number of service industry workers including those in the 'care' sector of nursing, nursing homes, social services, etc. The increasing proportion of elderly and very old frail people in the population (Wagstaff and Coakley, 1988) will increase 'care' demands, as can changes in medical practice, e.g. intensive care wards. There are also people whose needs are social as well as medical and those who, for psychological reasons, can be uncooperative, obstructive or violent, e.g. substance abusers in Accident and Emergency who provide a challenge to even the most experienced handler. Employees in the 'care' sector tend to be predominately female and may be particularly at risk because of the heavy social and occupational demands placed upon them in combining home and family duties with work.

Much of the heaviest work in manufacturing has been mechanized with the advent of fork-lift trucks, palletized loads, conveyors, etc. Until the 1950s, when this mechanization process really started to progress, 1 cwt or 50 kg was the standard packaged load handled by millions of workers, including women, during the 1939–45 World War, and most seemed unharmed by doing so. Today, such a load would be considered safe for a minority of workers and would be outside the safe capacity of the majority.

The manual content of most jobs, including housework, has also been reduced by the proliferation of small electrical hand tools, from electric drills and screwdrivers to food mixers. Increasingly, people drive to work and school rather than walk or cycle (Allied Dunbar, 1992), and stair climbing is replaced by escalators and lifts. School children are less physically active than earlier generations (Armstrong et al., 1990; Thirlaway and Benton, 1993).

These changes in the nature of work and in home and leisure activities have been accompanied by, and may have contributed towards, some of the changes in the working population. They are becoming heavier, fatter and taller. Most importantly they are less fit, both in a cardiovascular and muscular development sense. Many people have little experience of performing a wide range of physical tasks and are physically poorly equipped to do so. Their kinaesthetic sense may be poorly developed and they have no experience of the strategies that can be used to overcome difficult moving and handling situations.

Another aspect to consider is that trade unions and the media have widened people's understanding of their rights and employers' duties, and there seems to be an increasing willingness to sue when things go wrong. Even healthcare employees, who appear to be experts at making do and coping with a lack of, or poor, equipment and working environments, may be less willing to do so in the future. While OH physiotherapists will wish to support well-founded complaints based on management's failure to observe its legal duties and obligations, it is essential that they are perceived as being fair to both sides and take a balanced view. It is very tempting for individuals to blame work for all their problems, but their opinion may not be based on known medical facts and they may choose to ignore other contributory factors in their lifestyle or previous medical or employment history.

Legal issues and responsibilities

The Health and Safety at Work (HSW) Act (Health and Safety Executive, 1974) brought together earlier regulations and laid down duties on employers and employees to make work safer. A European Community Directive (Commission of the European Communities, 1990) and the present Manual Handling Operations Regulations (MHOR) (Health and Safety Executive, 1992a) have been in effect since January 1st 1993; these place primary duties on employers to:

1. Avoid hazardous manual handling operations where possible
2. Assess hazardous operations that cannot be avoided
3. Eliminate or reduce the risk of injury, using the assessment as a basis for action.

Section 2 of the HSW Act (1974), the MHOR (1992) and the Management of Health and Safety at Work Regulations (MHSWR) (Health and Safety Executive, 1992b) also lay duties on employers to provide training in safe techniques, and to given specific information and training on manual handling injury risk prevention to workers involved in manual handling tasks. Technique training should be secondary to ergonomic improvement and steps should be taken to optimize the design of manual handling operations and improve the task, load and working environment. Manual handling operations should be designed to suit individuals, and not the other way round (Health and Safety Executive, 1992b). Effective training should complement a safe system of work, not be used a substitute for it. The ultimate responsibility rests with management (see sections 37 and 40 HSW Act; Health and Safety Executive, 1974).

Section 7 of the HSW Act (1974) requires employees to take reasonable care for their own health and safety and that of others who may be affected by their activities and to co-operate with their employers to enable them to comply with their health and safety duties. They must follow safe systems of work as laid down by their employer (see regulation 5 of the MHOR; Health and Safety Executive, 1992a) and make use of appropriate equipment provided for them in accordance with such training and instruction given them by their employer (see regulation 12 of the MHSWR; Health and Safety Executive, 1992b). Employees also have a duty under the Reporting of Injuries, Diseases and Dangerous Occurrences Regulations (Health and Safety Executive, 1985) to report any sickness or injury where they are absent from work for 3 days or more. Such data are extremely useful in alerting the OH physiotherapist to possible problem work areas, as are clinical referrals.

Inanimate and animate loads

In handling inanimate objects it should always be possible to establish the characteristics of the load and the physical demands of the task before it is performed, although employees will need training to enable them to do so. Weight is only one of the factors to be considered and others such as size, stability and quality of grip may be of equal importance. In theory, every situation can be assessed, preplanned and made as easy and safe as possible. In practice, time pressures, lack of staff, poor packaging and lack of skill often mean that employees rush in without thinking and try to cope, with potentially dangerous consequences.

Animate loads (e.g. people) do not come in stock sizes or conditions. They may move, altering weight distribution and centre of gravity, and be unpredictable in the amount of assistance that is given or withheld. They can on occasion fight back and can suffer if inappropriately handled. Most importantly, people should be encouraged to help themselves as much as possible both for their own independence and the well-being of the healthcare employee. Where this is not possible, it must be remembered that humans feel pain and anxiety and need to have any procedure explained to them, e.g. the method of moving or any equipment being used; without this explanation the healthcare employee may not get the expected cooperation. Personal dignity needs to be preserved at all times and care taken if patients are connected to medical equipment which needs to be moved with them. For these reasons, assessment should be an integral part of the care plan and frequent updates may need to be made, taking into account the potential variables; failure to do this may cause injury to the healthcare employee, patient or both. Strategies may be needed, e.g. a controlled fall is often better for all concerned than trying to prevent a fall that is inevitable.

Time pressure, lack of staff, poor management, lack of skill and lack of equipment mean that employees often expose themselves to greater risks than are necessary. Training, practice, experience and a flexible approach are of great importance to a safe system of work when moving and handling loads, whether animate or inanimate.

Seating

Seating needs to be put into context within moving and handling. It may not be widely understood that sitting puts a greater compressive force on the spine than standing; therefore just standing up reduces pressure (Andersson, 1986). It follows that prolonged sitting even in a 'good' posture is stressful and in a 'bad' posture has potential for causing long-term damage. If lifting is carried out in a sitting position, particularly with the arms outstretched, e.g. lifting a heavy file off a shelf behind a desk, the mechanical forces involved are considerable. Many laboratory benches are made without kneeholes and workers have to sit with their knees facing sideways and their shoulders facing forward, which is very undesirable except for short periods, and standing or sit-standing is preferable.

Driving may be interspersed with loading and unloading, and studies show that the greater the number of hours spent in a motor vehicle, the higher the risk of back injury (Kelsey et al., 1984). Packaging and inspection workers, supermarket checkout and central sterile supply staff, among others, will all be handling goods from a seated position. If it is not possible to alter the height of the workstation, there will be wide differences in the relationship between employee and work surface, determined by the height of the employee. Employees will make postural adjustments to adjust to the misfit in order to carry out the task. These can be reduced by adjusting the height of the chair, although people are unlikely to do this unless they understand the reasons why they should do so, and the controls are extremely quick and simple to use, e.g. gas adjustable. When encouraged to do so, many employees on packaging lines and similar operations find that they can work more easily when standing up, since they have to lean forward, stretch and reach less. Work activities through a whole work shift must be taken into account and seating should be available for alternative working postures to be taken up if desired.

All employees need to understand why changing posture is good for the body and alternation between sitting and standing is recommended. Managers also need to understand why flexibility in working postures is necessary, so that they will not enforce rigid and unnecessary work practices.

Assessment of risk

Assessment which is so important in the OH context is a core skill of physiotherapists. Direct and regular observation of employees in their working environment and familiarity with actual loads, working conditions and practices are essential prerequisites when physiotherapists consider assessing risks or teaching others. Feedback from clinical work (where this is available) helps OH physiotherapists to weight the reality of risks and make more balanced judgements between perceived and actual risks.

Where a manual handling risk is identified, some guidance may need to be given to management as to the severity of the risk and the timespan in which it is reasonable to expect change. Even where management is committed to making work as safe as possible, many changes take time to implement and 'coping' behaviour may need to be used and taught in the interim period; this may be acceptable provided senior management's attention has been drawn (in writing) to the risk factors and the employees also understand that it is 'coping' techniques that they are learning and using.

In large organizations it may be more practical for the OH physiotherapist to have an input into the training of others, to make workplace assessments. In all areas, physiotherapists must be aware of the limitations of their knowledge and expertise and know when to call in other members of the team or outside experts. The more that high technology is employed in the working situation, the greater is the need for a multidisciplinary approach and the more care is needed not to remove one hazard and substitute another equally dangerous one. The OH physiotherapist should try to avoid being tied into one small part of an overall manual handling policy, i.e. training, and try to have an input at all levels; inability to do so has a potential to cause major problems, as well as frustration and lack of job satisfaction. Decisions may be taken by people with less relevant skills and experience and could result, for example, in the physiotherapist being required to train employees in a moving and handling task which requires them to use a piece of equipment which he/she regards as unsuitable and hazardous. Clinically, the physiotherapist could be treating numerous employees with injuries and problems arising from a work activity which had been assessed, in his/her view incorrectly, as without risk. Similarly, the physiotherapist could be teaching individual employees safe moving and handling techniques which go against a method which has been laid down in working procedures manuals.

An ergonomic approach involves assessing the task, load, environment and the individual employee's capability. There are a number of books and booklets on the market with suggested procedures. MHOR (Health and Safety Executive, 1992a) gives a useful baseline and can be adapted according to the particular activities of an individual organization. The features which may be responsible for foreseeable risks should be identified and attempts made to modify them.

The OH physiotherapists may pre-empt some of the problems likely to be exposed in an assessment by updating management and senior staff of new equipment and information. Staff should be encouraged to make the best use of the environment and be taught how to use the available equipment. Advice on matters concerning musculoskeletal problems, such as handling specific items or awkward or heavy patients, etc., may also be given on an *ad hoc* basis. Advice about ergonomics may be offered when work areas are upgraded, redesigned or re-equipped, or when new areas are designed, to ensure that they are complying with ergonomic principles. A copy of the relevant Health Building Note (Department of Health and Social Security and the Welsh Office, 1986) is useful and in a healthcare setting the introduction and explanation of the benefits of overhead hoists as an alternative to mobile ones is important. Any human performance deteriorates with repetition and tiredness and what may be easy at the start of a shift may be potentially damaging at the end.

Changes when risk is revealed

Where a workplace assessment reveals a manual handling risk, changes will be necessary and will fall into one or more of the categories described below.

Environmental changes

Avoidance of manual handling risk may lead to full mechanization by such equipment as fork-lift trucks, vacu-lifts, conveyor belts, hoists, etc., and where substantial and regular loads are moved in quantity this is the only satisfactory long-term solution. Reduction of manual handling risk may be achieved by the use of partial mechanization, such as the use of hand trucks or trolleys, rollers and other sliding systems, etc., or through changes to the structural layout. Care will be needed in the choice of equipment, and regular maintenance will need to be carried out. Any new equipment which is to be brought in as a result of the assessment process needs a trial prior to purchase. A hoist was purchased by management for a particular work area without prior consultation with, or trial by, the users or the lifting and handling adviser. It was subsequently found to be unsuitable and therefore unusable.

There is potential for serious mismatches to occur between the equipment chosen and the task it is supposed to carry out, particularly if the purchaser is not the user. Where there is a full and frank discussion of equipment on trial between managers and those who will be operators, there is less likelihood of problems in persuading employees to use what is provided, and less risk of injury because of misuse or inappropriate equipment. Training in safe and correct use of the equipment is necessary, and careful attention must be paid to problems of storage and access. Changes to the environment can have negative as well as positive effects and these must be considered before action is taken. Improving a floor surface to make it non-slip can reduce many moving and handling problems, because all lifting techniques require a secure and stable foot position. However, the resulting increase in friction and force needed to overcome inertia can make it more difficult to move trolleys or wheeled objects.

Changes in workplace layout

Simple changes can often reduce the need for moving or reduce its range, so lowering the risk involved. These can include where and how goods are stacked or stored and the removal or repositioning of objects or furniture which prevent easy and close access to the objects to be moved, e.g. moving beds, chairs, lockers or other obstacles in the work-place before any attempt is made to carry out the handling operation. Training has a major role in making employees aware of these strategies and how their use can reduce effort and risk.

Changes in the task

The task itself can be modified to reduce risk. The way that a load is packaged and the quality of the grip that an employee can get upon it has an enormous impact on the ease or difficulty with which it is handled. In industry, changing the packaging of larger, heavier or awkward items is not necessarily as difficulty or expensive as sometimes perceived, and strategies to improve grip and handling can be taught and applied, whether handling people or loads. The more compact the 'load' the easier it is to handle; small equipment, such as sliding devices for patients and detachable handles for loads, can make the task easier. Manual handling tasks that are acknowledged to be heavy should be alternated with lighter tasks to put less overall physiological load on the employee. Frequent, short rest periods will improve performance and lower musculoskeletal stress. Rotation of staff can have similar effects. Work is easier and safer if all employees are working as a team who appreciate each others' strengths and weaknesses. Training has an important role in encouraging tolerance and cooperation. There are many situations where one employee can 'set up' a dangerous situation for somebody else, e.g. putting a very heavy object on a high shelf, or leaving equipment where somebody else will fall over it, or not returning it to the correct place so that it cannot be found when next required. Any new work processes or equipment brought in as a result of an assessment process should be monitored. Another example is given where provision of hoists in a work area did reduce back injuries as planned, but because the lifting mechanism was hand pumped, shoulder injuries and complaints started to increase; one problem had been eliminated only to be replaced by another. (The hoists now used are push button and battery operated.)

Changes in management attitudes

Managers' attitudes may need to change. They must be encouraged to pay attention to any manual handling problems that workers raise with them and not to dismiss them as coming from troublemakers or 'fusspots'. They may need educating into taking a flexible approach which takes account of individual employees' strengths and weaknesses, both mental and physical. For example, use of temporary or permanent work restrictions can enable workers with problems to continue work safely, albeit in a limited capacity (Dean and Congdon, 1984) and these can have very positive effects in reducing sickness absence. They improve morale and are a useful part of a rehabilitation regime. Similarly, as people age, their muscle strength, flexibility and speed decline, but this is usually offset by a more responsible attitude which leads the employee to think and plan before acting and to acknowledge when a task is beyond his or her capabilities.

Training in manual handling emphasizes the need to think, assess and plan. Employees with severe problems in their personal lives or in work relationships often do not have their minds on their jobs and can therefore be a danger to themselves and others. It should be recognized that they must be watched and supervised more closely than normal. Any employee reporting for work who is obviously unwell should be sent to the OH department for assessment before being allowed to work. An injury sustained at home or playing sport can severely compromise handling ability, as can more general illness. A further injury may then arise at work which was preventable.

The manager or supervisor has a major role to play in team building and encouraging good cooperation between workers in handling tasks, enforcing safe working practices and identifying individual workers experiencing problems with a manual task. Where manual handling tasks are made as easy, efficient and safe as possible, there is often a substantial reduction in damage to the load and time spent moving it, resulting in less wastage, better quality and higher productivity. Good practice has economic benefits which can more than outweigh the costs. The OH physiotherapist can play a key role in facilitating and supporting these changes.

Changes in employee attitudes

Employees as well as managers may need to change their attitudes. We all tend to become very set in our patterns of behaviour and continue doing things the same old way quite regardless of changes all around us. When it comes to manual handling skills very few long-term employees will see themselves as having any need to learn anything, or to change their behaviour, and may actively resent being asked to do so.

Frequent visits from the OH physiotherapist to a work area can build confidence among employees, indicating that their real work and problems are understood and so help to soften attitudes. Specific attitude problems identified should be aired and discussed in training sessions.

Training programmes

Managers need to be fully aware of current legislation and should be prepared to offer necessary facilities, venue, equipment and time. With regard to training, it is up to management to enable staff to attend training sessions and up to the staff to ensure that they attend. Physiotherapists in OH must be familiar with the HSW Act and all relevant regulations and keep up to date with any changes. Accurate records of training programmes are essential; see *Moving and Handling Factsheets* (1992) and *Standards for Trainers in Moving and Handling* (1993) (Chartered Society of Physiotherapy).

Aims and objectives

The overall aim of a training programme is to reduce the incidence of musculoskeletal problems from moving and handling and poor and sustained working postures.

The general objectives of training programmes are to:

1. Explain current legislation and the responsibilities of the employer and employee
2. Explain the nature and meaning of musculoskeletal problems and suggest why musculoskeletal statistics seem to be rising
3. Teach the concept of body awareness and individual capabilities
4. Identify a process for assessing the task and the load and ways to reduce any risks by trying to improve ergonomic aspects of the situation
5. Explain and identify a 'safe system of work' in relation to the trainees' work area

6. Give technique training, including the safe use of equipment
7. Teach strategies for overcoming difficult moving and handling situations, e.g. breaking the load into smaller sections, staged lifts, reduction of friction
8. Make people more aware of lifestyle factors and the risks of fatigue and cumulative stress
9. Enable the trainees to relate all the above to themselves and their working situation
10. Encourage group discussion of moving and handling problems in the work area and ways that could be used to try to overcome them.

Further objectives for training in patient handling are to ensure that the healthcare worker can demonstrate an ability to:

1. Communicate with the patient/client – this may be verbal, written, by demonstration or by touch – and communicate with fellow workers
2. Encourage the patients/clients to move for themselves
3. Use available equipment
4. Choose the correct manual handling technique where necessary, in the context of the characteristics of the patient and any colleague who may help.

Preparing for training

Before any attempt is made to organize moving and handling training, OH physiotherapists must visit the department to be trained so that they are totally familiar with all the work that goes on there, the containers and equipment used, and the management and supervisory style. Certain key facts must be established, such as whether it is to be part of a routine training programme or whether training has been requested because there has been an accident or there is a recognized problem. There is often a hidden agenda in requests for training and it is important to try to determine what it is.

It is important to establish whether all the workers or only new employees in an area are to be trained. If the latter – is there a large turnover of employees and, if so, why? Since the emphasis on training should be on teamwork and group safety, all the employees in an area or ward should be trained together and there is every reason to repeat training that may not have been fully absorbed on the first occasion.

An appraisal of the supervisors should be made. Have they been trained and do they accept what is taught and the time required to teach and practise it? Do they reinforce the training day by day? In the past, training has often been a quick video following by an hour or so of practice. Is it possible for someone to watch a video of a sport (e.g. tennis) and then go out and play the game? An aspiring tennis player needs a certain level of fitness and co-ordination, to be taught the strokes and to practise. So it is with moving and handling trainees, and the OH physiotherapist has to be assertive in making this clear. Supervisors must have a realistic understanding of the breadth and depth of training necessary for employees to become competent in moving and handling. If supervisors are not fully supportive of what is taught, training is unlikely to succeed. Every attempt should be made by the trainer to listen to and understand and supervisors' problems. The trainer may wish to modify what is taught in the light of their comments or to support the supervisors in pressing management for changes to be made in working practice or equipment.

Any specific hazards or tasks that are thought to be particularly difficult should be identified. Have these been revealed through workplace assessment or are they already known to management and have they any plans to remedy the problem other than by training? For example, there may be too little space to use or to manoeuvre equipment. It must be made clear to the requesting management that no amount of safe training can overcome such hazards and make an unsafe system safe.

The aspects of the present behaviour of employees which the trainer wishes to change should be carefully considered, e.g. whether there is any problem with their general attitude towards safety or other workers, or if there is a lack of teamwork. The task demands, the work organization and the actual techniques used to move and handle loads should all be analysed to determine how training can be structured and how to increase trainees' understanding of the need for change and to motivate them towards achieving this.

Training sessions

If it is not possible to train everybody at once, training should be targeted towards staff most likely to be able to influence others, and staff identified to be most at risk. Staff at risk may be employees returning after injury or illness, for whom a training update is strongly recommended. Staff with problems (whether work related or not) also need to be monitored regularly and may need individual assessment and training.

It is extremely helpful if line managers or supervisors or clinical managers attend the training sessions and take part in the discussions; it shows that they regard the training and its implementation as important and they are in a position to set an agenda for change. Close liaison with safety officers and their participation in training sessions can also be very beneficial. They should be in a position to monitor changes and liaise regularly with management and, above all, they are aware of other hazards and constraints and can add their knowledge and expertise.

It is not possible to assume a base level of knowledge in trainees. It is better to start with a period of revision to ascertain previous knowledge, skills, attitude and understanding and then build on this. Teaching methods will need to be adjusted to the audience, e.g. within the health service with its enormous ethnic mix it is very likely that there will be people who are unable to read or write more than their name in English. There is little point in showing written overheads in such cases and better by far to use diagrams, role play, video and practical techniques. Some people of ethnic groups do not like to touch or work with the opposite sex; others do not like to feel that they are issuing orders when telling a patient how to move.

Training given must reflect the actual work done in the workplace and should be followed up by further training and

supervision in the workplace, ideally by the OH physiotherapist or a senior member of staff who has further training in
order to carry out this training and supervisory role. Understanding all aspects of the work situation of the trainees
should enable a trainer to tailor the training to their specific
needs. Practical technique must be taught using the containers and/or equipment that the trainees use and in conditions as similar as possible. Trainees must appreciate that
every individual has his/her own safe capacity in what he or
she can move or handle and must live within its confines.
Some individuals are naturally stronger and better co-ordin-
ated than others and no amount of training can change this
fact. Using good techniques cannot enable a person to lift
more weight; it can only reduce the amount of effort needed,
and put less stress on the body and lessen the chance of
injury.

Individuals cannot decide whether a task is within or
outside their capacity until they understand the nature of the
load. Its size and shape are visibly obvious but not it weight,
stability or centre of gravity. There are particular difficulties
with opaque containers of fluid, which when partially full
present unanticipated changes in the centre of gravity. Most
techniques of inanimate load assessment thus involve turning, tipping slightly, or rocking. Strategies for reducing effort
and making moving and handling easier also need to be
taught.

Healthcare workers, patients and their families must be
educated to understand that it is in the best interests of all
concerned to enable the patient to maintain maximal independence. It is possible to care without necessarily assisting
physically; this is a concept to which nurses and carers are
slowly coming round. If, as a result of training, patients
requiring assistance are handled better, i.e. more comfort-
ably, there is a hidden benefit in that they will respond better,
sleep better and in the long term will require less help from
their carer. Training will be needed in manual handling
techniques and in how to cope during emergency situations,
such as dealing with the patient who falls in a confined space.

Training must involve trainees as actively as possible,
encouraging and stimulating discussion and participation.

Some trainees may already have skills and strategies for overcoming difficult handling situations which they can be encouraged to share, and the trainers may also learn new techniques or strategies in the process. Difficulties and obstacles must be explored and possible ways of overcoming them discussed. Where a consensus of agreement for the need for change and the method to be tried exists, it is likely that doubters will gradually be drawn in by peer pressure and a wish to conform.

Why training programmes may fail

Training can and does fail both within industry and the health service for a number of reasons.

1. The most common reason for failure of training is that the aims which it sought to achieve were unrealistic; training is an inappropriate solution to a problem which needs to be solved by ergonomic or task organization changes. Managers tend to see training as a quick, easy solution to problems which places the onus for change on the employees rather than on them. Blame can then be apportioned – 'you didn't lift correctly' – instead of an acceptance that the task could be making unreasonable or excessive physical demands. Although this goes against the spirit and word of the recent legislation, it will be with reluctance that some managers accept the need for structural and ergonomic changes, with their higher cost implications.
2. Ergonomic changes do not necessarily cost money, e.g. changes in task or workplace layout. Where structural change is necessary, there may be an acute shortage of funds available to managers to make changes. Complex problems will only yield to a multifaceted and sustained team approach and if no ergonomic improvements are made, all the worker ends up with is an update in technique training and coping strategies which are known to be ineffective.
3. Further training may be needed where major changes of function, equipment or staff occur in the work area, e.g.

a change in manufacturing process or containers, a change in staffing levels on a surgical ward converted to elderly care usage.
4. Training can also fail if the actual techniques taught are not correct, e.g. there is as yet no consensus of opinion as to how far the knees should bend when performing a lift, or whether the entire surface of both feet should remain on the ground throughout. More than one technique of moving a specific load may be needed in order to accommodate differing sizes of workers.
5. Staff and management may continue to follow the custom and practice of many years of manual handling techniques only and fail to support, encourage and reinforce the use of equipment and procedures as taught in training.
6. Trainees may fail to absorb training as a result of poor facilities, poor teaching techniques, poor presentation skills or a lack of sufficient time.
7. Training may fail to achieve change in employees' attitudes because they do not accept the relevance of training to their work or see any need to change their behaviour. It is thought that knowledge will not be translated into behaviour change unless there is modification of attitudes and beliefs. Mature employees who know and fully appreciate the importance of care of their body may be less likely to rush in and do the task without stopping to think and assess if there are time pressures to move a load or complete a ward routine.
8. Present economic conditions tend to pressure fewer employees to do more work. The resulting mental and physical fatigue can result in employees not making the effort to set up and prepare a task properly and safely as taught.

Monitoring and evaluation

It is particularly difficult to monitor moving and handling as sickness absence is so multifactorial (Artus, 1993; Howard, 1993). In addition, even when epidemiological data are available there may be under-reporting which can give false perceptions. Equally, accident statistics can be misleading because when awareness is raised by legislation or training, there is a tendency to record very trivial incidents and numbers appear to rise. It can be difficult to make time to go into the workplace to monitor changes and evaluate courses and outcomes. It is important to do so, and feedback may be received which will encourage trainers to modify course content or presentation. What is wanted is a demonstration of transfer of knowledge and skill into the workplace away from continuous supervision; for this, it is necessary for the OH physiotherapist to either visit the workplace unannounced and observe work activities and postures, or to have a supervisor in the workplace trained to assess. Checks will have to be made to ensure that they continue to fill this role. It may also be useful to monitor the number of times a piece of equipment, such as a hoist, is used in a given period of time.

It is important to note that more and more advice is being sought from OH physiotherapists in compensation cases for plaintiff or defendant. For this reason it is essential to maintain accurate records of the content of training and to be aware of other current strategies in the organization. It is also helpful to keep out-of-date books and training videos as a reminder of what was then thought to be acceptable practice.

The role of the OH physiotherapist in moving and handling issues can be challenging and fulfilling and have a long-term influence on the health and well-being of all employees. It needs support from all levels of management within the organization. Without this support, the role is likely to be frustrating, unsatisfactory and ultimately unsuccessful. Support must be more than verbal platitudes or a grudging acceptance of legal requirements. It needs to be a sustained commitment to improving working methods and practices, improving management in the workplace, and increasing the skill and knowledge of employees. A team approach, with sharing of ideas and experience and a willingness to listen and learn, at all levels, makes a positive outcome more likely.

References

Allied Dunbar (1992) *National Fitness Survey*, Health Education Authority and Sports Council, London

Andersson, G.B.J. (1986) Loads on the spine during sitting. In *Ergonomics of Working Posture* (eds N. Corlett and J. Wilson). Taylor and Francis, London

Armstrong, N., Balding, J., Gentle, P. and Kirby, B. (1990) Patterns of physical activity among 11 to 16 year old British children. *British Medical Journal*, **301**, 203–205

Artus, K. (1993) Attendance and absence control; whose responsibility? *Occupational Health*, **45**, 95–96

Chartered Society of Physiotherapy (1992) *Moving and Handling Factsheets 9* and *9A*, CSP, Bedford Row, London

Chartered Society of Physiotherapy (1993) *Standards of Physiotherapy Practice for Trainers in Moving and Handling*, CSP, Bedford Row, London

Commission of the European Communities (1990) Council directive on the minimum health and safety requirements for the manual handling of loads where there is a risk particularly of back injury to workers. Fourth individual directive within the meaning of article 16(1) of directive 89/391/EEC, 90/269/EEC. *Official Journal of the European Communities* 21.6.90 no. **1**, Brussels, pp. 156/9–13

Dean, S.P. and Congdon, G.J. (1984) Rehabilitation after illness and injury – a study of temporary alternative work arrangements. *Journal of the Society of Occupation Medicine*, **34**, 46–49

Employment Gazette (1993) Employment workforce. Jan, pp. 8–10

Genaidy, A.M., Karwowski, W., Guo, L., Hidalgo, J. and Garbutt, G. (1992) Physical training: a tool for increasing work tolerance limits of employees engaged in manual handling tasks. *Ergonomics*, **35**, 1081–1102

Health and Safety Commission (1991) *Manual Handling of Loads. Proposals for Regulations and Guidance*, Sir Robert Jones Workshops, Units 3 and 5–9, Grain Industries Estate, Harlow St., Liverpool

Health and Safety Executive (1974) *Health and Safety at Work Act*, HMSO, London

Health and Safety Executive (1985) *Reporting of Injuries, Diseases and Dangerous Occurrences Regulations*, HMSO, London

Health and Safety Executive (1992a) *Manual Handling Regulations and Guidance*, HMSO, London

Health and Safety Executive (1992b) *Management of Health and Safety at Work Regulations and Approved Code of Practice*, HMSO, London

Department of Health and Social Security and the Welsh Office (1986) Health Building Note 40. *Common Activity Spaces*, vol. 1, HMSO, London

Howard, G. (1993) Malingering; a fraudulent issue. *Occupational Health*, **45**, 98–100

Kelsey, J. L., Githens, P. B., O'Connor, T. (1984) Acute prolapsed lumbar intervertebral disc. *Spine*, **9**, 608–613

McKenzie, R. A. (1983) *The Lumbar Spine and Back Pain: Mechanical Diagnosis and Therapy*, Spinal Publications, Waikanae, Wellington, New Zealand

National Back Pain Association and Royal College of Nursing (1993) *The Guide to Handling Patients*, 3rd edn, NBPA, London

Thirlaway, K. and Benton, D. (1993) Physical activity in primary- and secondary-school children in West Glamorgan. *Health Education Journal*, **52**, 37–41

Wagstaff, P. and Coakley, D. (1988) *Physiotherapy and The Elderly Patient*, Croom Helm, London

Chapter 12

Prevention and treatment of upper limb disorders

Jeffrey D. Boyling

Introduction

The last decade has seen an increase in the number of individuals with musculoskeletal conditions affecting the upper limbs. These conditions, known as 'upper limb disorders' in the UK, have been decribed by various terms in the UK and other countries. These problems have been the subject of numerous books and conferences (Buckle, 1987; Stevenson, 1987; Bullock, 1990; Barton et al., 1992; Hagberg and Kilbom, 1992). Despite the proliferation of information, confusion caused by terminology as well as confusion amongst those involved in the examination and treatment of those affected has added to the problem of managing these musculoskeletal conditions. Much money has been spent by companies and individuals on treatment as well as finding ergonomic solutions. Cases have gone to court and there has been associated media attention. It has become a growth industry and yet for many individuals the mystery of the problem remains unexplained. This should not be the case. The application of ergonomics can prevent upper limb disorders. However, for those cases that do occur, early reporting and specific treatment based on careful clinical examination can lead to recovery and return to work.

What is an upper limb disorder?

To answer the question of what is an upper limb disorder, it is necessary to look at the terminology used: Table 12.1 shows numerous descriptive terms which are used and which apply to the same thing. Definitions have been given for some of these terms. In 1985 the National Occupational Health and Safety Commission (NOHSC) in Australia defined repetitive strain injury (RSI) as: 'a soft tissue disorder caused by the overloading of particular muscle groups from repeated use or maintenance of constrained postures. It occurs among workers performing tasks involving either frequent repetitive movements of the limbs or the maintenance of fixed postures for prolonged periods, for example process workers, keyboard operators and machinists' (NOHSC, 1985). In 1986 the same group issued a revised definition which stated that RSI was 'a collective term for a range of conditions characterised by discomfort or persistent pain in muscles, tendons and other soft tissues, with or without physical manifestations' (NOHSC, 1986i). This definition also acknowledged the fact that 'some conditions which fall within the scope of Repetition Strain Injury are well defined and understood medically, but many are not, and the basis for their cause and development is yet to be determined'. Four years later, the Health and Safety Executive (HSE) in the UK (HSE, 1990) considered upper limb disorders to 'encompass a range of conditions affecting the soft tissues of the hand, wrist, arm and shoulder'.

Table 12.1 Descriptive terms for upper limb disorders

Term	Abbreviation	Country
Repetitive strain injury	RSI	Australia
Repetitive motion injury	RMI	Canada
Cumulative trauma disorder	CTD	United States
Occupational cervicobrachial disorder	OCD	Sweden, Japan
Occupational overuse disorder	OOD	Australia

The problem with these terms and definitions is that they do not give any clear indication as to the structure(s) causing the problem. Ranney (1993) stated that they are statements of causation. Even so, in terms of the mechanisms suggested, they may be misleading. They are umbrella terms to cover what can be an ill-defined symptom complex. However, upper limb disorders are often considered to be in the hand and forearm, and other terms such as those listed in Table 12.2 are frequently used. These terms are diagnostic labels for clearly-defined clinical conditions.

Table 12.2 Diagnostic terms used for upper limb disorders

Carpal tunnel syndrome	Compression neuropathy
Tendinitis	Tenosynovitis
Lateral epicondylitis	Medial epicondylitis
Bursitis	De Quervain's

Pheasant (1991) has classified these musculoskeletal conditions as follows: synonymous generic terms, specific clinical conditions, less specific clinical conditions and occupational variants. Nevertheless, each one of the descriptive, diagnostic and occupational terms will have a set of symptoms and signs. In each case these will vary from patient to patient and in each patient the symptoms and signs may change from day to day. Various symptoms have been reported for upper limb disorders including discomfort, aching, pains, paraesthesia, anaesthesia, heaviness, swelling/fullness and burning. These symptoms can be reported in the conditions already shown in Tables 12.1 and 12.2 as well as in other conditions which are not listed. This leads to an important point in the management of upper limb disorders: people with the above symptoms should not be labelled as having an upper limb disorder until a thorough medical examination has been conducted. This is important because one of the problems with upper limb disorders is the unnecessary anxiety that can be created by inappropriate use of terms. This same anxiety is not associated with spinal pain. Therefore, a key element in the overall management is a thorough examination of any individual with symptoms, so as to establish an accurate diagnosis. This is where physical therapists need to continually update their skills to keep abreast of the latest knowledge (see Butler, 1991).

In summary, upper limb disorder is used as a collective term for those conditions characterized by discomfort or persistent pain in muscles, tendons and other soft tissues. This means an 'upper limb disorder' can be a clearly-defined clinical condition or an ill-defined symptom complex. However, in the interests of the patient, precise clinical diagnoses should be used and the term upper limb disorder reserved for the group of patients with an ill-defined complex of symptoms. Fortunately, the application of ergonomics to prevent the pain of upper limb disorders should not be affected by terminology.

Prevention

To prevent upper limb disorders it is necessary to be aware of the risk factors. Numerous authors have listed various risk factors, as shown in Table 12.3. Non-occupational factors can also be associated with upper limb disorders.

Prevention also requires tools so that examination of the workplace can be undertaken. In the UK guidance has been produced by the Health and Safety Executive. This covers a general publication on the work-related upper limb disorders (HSE, 1990) as well as the use of display screen equipment (HSE, 1992). The former is geared to the non-office environment. However, none of these is quantitative in approach.

Rapid upper limb assessment (RULA)

RULA, a rapid upper limb assessment developed by McAtamney and Corlett (1992, 1993) is a method which looks at the physical aspects of the work; it does not consider the environmental aspects such as temperature and lighting, nor does it evaluate the component due to stress. To date, no system has been developed to assess all factors liable to

Table 12.3 Risk factors in the production of upper limb disorders

Risk factor	Author
Frequency of repetitive notions	Brown, 1983
Force used in performing movements	
Duration of work without rest	
Degree of static muscle loading of trunk and shoulders in maintaining a fixed posture	
Individual capacity for such work	
Faults in workplace, job design and equipment	
Bonus and overtime incentives to increase productivity	
Psychological or emotional stress leading to excessive muscle loading and ergonomic inefficiency	
Biomechanical factors	NOHSC, 1985
Faulty work organization	
Deficiencies in personnel practices	
Personal	McPhee, 1983
Social	
Environmental	
Force	Putz-Anderson, 1988
Repetition	
Posture	
No rest	
Fixed or constrained body positions	Bertolini and
Continual repetition of movements	Drewczynski, 1990
Force concentrated on small parts of the body such as the hand or wrist	
A pace of work that does not allow sufficient recovery between movements	

NOHSC, National Occupational Health and Safety Commission (Australia).

contribute to an upper limb disorder. However, RULA is an excellent starting point.

RULA involves a number of stages. These cover simple postural assessments for the following body segments: upper arms; lower arms; wrist; neck; trunk and legs. For example, the upper arm is scored on the degrees of extension/flexion as well as shoulder elevation and abduction. For the upper limb and the trunk/legs a component is added for muscle use as well as for force or load. Each of these items is scored and the resulting score gives the user a risk rating. This will give the user objective information on what action should be taken, ranging from no action because the result is satisfactory or immediate investigation and action to rectify the problem. The system (McAtamney and Corlett 1993) has been validated and tested for reliability, which is important when reporting to management. The other aspect worth noting is that it is easy to apply so it can be taught to workplace managers and supervisors in order to develop in-house expertise.

Education

The other aspect to prevention is education of the workforce in basic ergonomics. Managers need to be aware of the risk factors listed in Table 12.3 as well as ergonomics. This covers anatomy, anthropometry, biomechanics, work physiology, environmental physiology and psychology. For the worker, ergonomic training places greater emphasis on the physical aspects of the task.

Workers therefore need to be aware of some key principles. With respect to anatomy, key principles include adopting balanced joint positions, avoiding static muscle work and avoiding nerve compression. Reversal of posture is also important in those tasks where postural variation is not great. The work of Gore and Tasker (1988) is helpful in this matter. Lee et al. (1992) have reviewed exercises for visual display terminal (VDT) operators but have failed to appreciate the postures which may contribute to clinical conditions. However, their suggestion that greater attention to both the practical and therapeutic aspects of exercises for VDT operators is needed is correct. Staff also need to be aware of the importance of early reporting should problems such as musculoskeletal discomfort occur; this facilitates the management of any musculoskeletal problem.

Management

While prevention by attention to the risk factors listed in Table 12.4 needs continual emphasis, cases of upper limb disorders may still occur. Then the management of the upper limb disorder is dependent on a number of factors. There must be early reporting of any musculoskeletal symptoms. Medical opinion should be sought. Where necessary, early treatment should be commenced. The flowcharts in the Australian Code of Practice (NOHSC, 1986ii) are designed to

Table 12.4   Risk factor awareness for managers

Risk factor for upper limb disorders

Awkward, rigid or sustained working positions
Bonus and piece-rate systems
Changes in the work process
Compulsory overtime
Excessive work rates
Inadequate rest breaks
Inadequate training
Knock or blow to a vulnerable area
Lack of control over the work process
Lack of job variation
Monitoring of work rate by machine
Overbearing supervision
Poor visual display unit workstation design and layout
Poor workplace, tool or equipment design
Poorly-maintained equipment
Rapid repetitive movements
Returning to work from holiday or illness
Speeding up of process or production lines
Vibration
Work involving twisting, gripping or overstretching

help direct individuals and managers in the right direction with regard to resolving problems. It should be noted that management covers both treatment and assessment of the risk factors in the workplace which may have resulted in a musculoskeletal problem: the NOHSC flowcharts reinforce this point. Codes of practice and legislation have been implemented by a number of countries to help employers and employees reduce the toll of upper limb disorders.

Treatment

The aim of treatment is to restore to normal function those tissues which are not normal. This is dependent on a thorough and accurate examination. It is important that clinical reasoning (Jones, 1994) is utilized to the maximum in sorting out the multiple symptoms which are sometimes reported. This approach makes full use of the Maitland (1986, 1991) approach to assessment. However, two specific areas warrant mention when dealing with upper limb disorders: the first concerns the role of neural tissue, while the second is muscle imbalance.

Pioneering work by Maitland (1978) and Elvey (1979) has focused attention on the neural tissue as a source of symptoms as well as a factor in the limitation of normal movement. In relation to upper limb disorders the work of Elvey was expanded by Kenneally (1985) but the major advance has been made by Butler (1991). Butler has developed the original examination concept to the point where the individual nerves in the upper limb can be selectively tested for movement and symptom production; this has lead to a better understanding of symptom production and variation in upper limb disorders. The work of Elvey et al. (1986) as well as Quintner and Elvey (1991) on the neurogenic basis of RSI should not go unreported.

Muscle imbalance is not a new area. Kendall et al. (1971) led the field in this area and subsequent work by Janda (1983) and Sahrmann (1993, personal communication) has developed it further. However, in the chronic cases referred for treatment there is a role for the correction of muscle imbalance. Persistent symptoms may be due to muscle tension irritating neural tissue. Thus the examination should note any muscle imbalance.

Other specific aspects in the treatment of upper limb disorders need to be noted. First, it is essential that the patient has a clear understanding of what tissues have been affected. This is part of the rehabilitation process because patients need to know what they can and cannot do. An understanding of the tissue mechanics, particularly when neural tissue is involved, is of importance. Second, depending on severity and irritability of tissues it is important that the patient appreciates the role of rest and activity. Rest (i.e. no movement) is the standard prescription to relieve pain but can be counter-productive in cases of upper limb disorders. In the vast majority of cases the risk factor of a static posture has been present in the work performed by the person. In other words, there has been no movement and prolonging this state is not compatible with recovery. Splinting is sometimes used to rest those parts where symptoms are experienced. This can result in exacerbation of the patient's condition. The compression of the splint may affect the normal function of local blood and nerve tissue. Therefore, it is recommended that splinting is not used.

Fear may need to be overcome and this is where a gradual re-introduction of activity is necessary. Frequently, patients will try to do too much too soon and suffer a 'flare-up'. This is just a reaction and should not be considered as different from any other musculoskeletal reaction; for example, ankle stiffness due to increased swelling brought about by increased weight-bearing/walking postankle sprain is a reaction and will settle if dealt with correctly: the same applies to upper limb disorders.

Another aspect worth noting, particularly in the chronic cases, is the role of the sympathetic nervous system; Butler (1991) discussed this and its role is worth remembering in those cases with swelling, blanching and temperature changes in the hands. The autonomic nervous system needs to be considered in mechanical terms and as such there are techniques for its examination. Attention to anatomy will indicate that the tests will vary from that for a spinal cord by virtue of the lateral location of the sympathetic chains. Trunk lateral flexion, rotation and mobilization over the rib attachments are required in treatment.

Naturally, with chronic cases conditioning is often required to restore a level of fitness suitable for return to the workplace. It is preferable to maintain the individual in the workplace if suitable tasks can be found. However, in those cases where sick leave has been taken, a graduated return to the workplace is advocated. For any return to be successful there must be a commitment from all parties: management, medical and employee. Changes to the workplace to eliminate risk factors need to be undertaken prior to this stage.

Prognosis

With regard to prognosis, patients will fall into three categories. The first group will achieve full recovery and return to work. The second group will be symptom- and sign-free but when back in the workplace will experience a return of symptoms. The possible reasons for this include a failure to modify the workplace according to ergonomic principles (see Grandjean 1982; Pheasant 1986), or a sensitivity still present in the tissues treated, especially neural tissue. There have been and will be cases where intervention has taken place too late and unfortunately a small number of individuals will fill the third category. The prognosis for those individuals will not include full recovery and return to work. These individuals will be left with persistent pain which may preclude them from work completely. Cohen et al. (1992) has discussed the problem of refractory cervicobrachial pain. This third category area needs further research but the work of Gibson et al. (1991) and Helme et al. (1992) has highlighted the fact that the chronic pain reported by RSI patients is associated with organic pathophysiology which affects local pain pathways.

Conclusion

Upper limb disorders are preventable and the application of ergonomics can achieve this. However, should an individual unwittingly sustain an upper limb disorder, it is treatable. Early effective treatment based on sound examination procedures and clinical reasoning is essential, otherwise a chronic problem can develop. Unfortunately recovery from any chronic condition, musculoskeletal or otherwise, is not always possible. This reinforces the need for greater emphasis on prevention and early reporting of musculoskeletal symptoms.

References

Barton, N. J., Hooper, G., Noble, J. and Steel, W. M. (1992) Occupational causes of disorders in the upper limb. *British Medical Journal*, **304**, 309–311

Bertolini, R. and Drewczynski, A. (1990) *Repetitive Motion Injuries*, Canadian Centre for Occupational Health and Safety, Ontario

Brown, C. (1983) An overview on diagnosis and management. In *Proceedings of Seminar on Repetition Strain Injuries* (Sydney, 1983), Arthritis and Rheumatism Council, Sydney, pp. 1–8

Buckle, P. (1987) *Musculoskeletal Disorders at Work*, Taylor and Francis, London

Bullock, M. I. (1990) *Ergonomics; The Physiotherapist in the Workplace*, Churchill Livingstone, Edinburgh.

Butler, D. (1991) *Mobilisation of the Nervous System*, Churchill Livingstone, Edinburgh

Cohen, M. L., Arroyo, J. F., Champion, G. D. and Browne, C. D. (1992) In search of the pathogenesis of refactory cervicobrachial pain syndrome, *Medical Journal of Australia*, **156**, 432–436

Elvey, R. L. (1979) Brachial plexus tension tests for the pathoanatomical origin of arm pain. In *Aspects of Manipulative Therapy*, Lincoln Institute of Health Services, Melbourne, Australia, pp. 105–110

Elvey, R., Quinter, J. L. and Thomas, A. N. (1986) A clinical study of RSI. *Australian Family Physician*, **15**, 1314–1315, 1319, 1322

Gibson, S. J., Le Vasseur, S. A. and Helme, R. D. (1991) Cerebral event-related responses induced by CO_2 laser stimulation in subjects suffering from cervico-brachial syndrome. *Pain*, **47**, 173–182

Gore, A. and Tasker, D. (1988) *Pause Gymnastics*, CCH Australia, Sydney

Grandjean, E. (1982) *Fitting the Task to the Man*, Taylor and Francis, London

Hagberg, M. and Kilbom, A. (1992) *International Scientific Conference on Prevention of Work-Related Musculoskeletal Disorders*, PREMUS, National Institute of Occupational Health, Sweden

Health and Safety Executive (1990) *Work Related Upper Limb Disorders: A Guide to Prevention*, HMSO, London

Health and Safety Executive (1992) *Display Screen Equipment Work: Guidance on Regulation*, HMSO, London

Helme, R. D., Le Vasseur, S. A. and Gibson, S. J. (1992) RSI revisited: evidence for psychological and physiological differences from an age, sex and occupation matched control group. *Australian and New Zealand Journal of Medicine*, **22**, 23–29

Janda, V. (1983) *Muscle Function Testing*, Butterworths, London

Jones, M. A. (1994) Clinical reasoning process in manipulative therapy. In *Grieve's Modern Manual Therapy*, 2nd edn (eds J. D. Boyling and N. Palastanga), Churchill Livingstone, Edinburgh, Chapter 34

Kendall, H. O., Kendall, F. P. and Wadsworth, G. E. (1971) *Muscles Testing and Function*, 2nd edn, Williams and Wilkins, Baltimore

Kenneally, M. (1985) The upper limb tension test. In *Proceedings, Manipulative Therapists Association of Australia, 4th Biennial Conference* (Brisbane, 1985), pp.259–273

Lee, K., Swanson, N., Sauter, S., Wickstrom, R., Waikar, A. and Mangum, M. (1992) A review of exercises recommended for VDT operators. *Applied Ergonomics*, **23**, 387–408

Maitland, G. D. (1978) Movement of pain sensitive structures in the vertebral canal in a group of physiotherapy students. In *Proceedings of Inaugural Congress of Manipulative Therapists Association of Australia* (Sydney, 1978). Manipulative Therapists Association of Australia, Sydney, Australia

Maitland, G. D. (1986) *Vertebral Manipulation*, 5th edn, Butterworths, London

Maitland, G. D. (1991) *Peripheral Manipulation*, 3rd edn, Butterworth–Heinemann, London

McAtamney, L. and Corlett, E. N. (1992) *Reducing the Risks of Work Related Upper Limb Disorders: A Guide and Methods*, Institute for Occupational Ergonomics, University of Nottingham

McAtamney, L. and Corlett, E. N. (1993) RULA: a survey method for the investigation of work-related upper limb disorders. *Applied Ergonomics*, **24**, pp. 91–99

McPhee, B. (1987) The mechanism of repetition strains. In *Readings in RSI* (ed. M. Stevenson), New South Wales University Press, Sydney, pp. 40–46

National Occupational Health and Safety Commission (1985) *Interim Report of the RSI Committee*, Australian Government Printing Service, Canberra, p. vi

National Occupational Health and Safety Commission (1986) *Repetition Strain Injury: A Report and Model Code of Practice*, Australian Government Printing Service, Canberra, (i) p. x; (ii) pp. 61–63

Pheasant, S. (1986) *Bodyspace: Anthropometry, Ergonomics and Design*, Taylor and Francis, London

Pheasant, S. (1991) *Ergonomics, Work and Health*, Macmillan Press, Basingstoke

Putz-Anderson, V. (1988) *Cumulative Trauma Disorders: A Manual for Musculoskeletal Diseases of the Upper Limbs*, Taylor and Francis, London

Quinter, J. and Elvey, R. (1991) *The Neurogenic Hypothesis of RSI*, Working Paper 24 (ed. G. Bammer), National Centre for Epidemiology and Population Health, Australian National University, Canberra

Ranney, D. (1993) Work related chronic injuries of the forearm and hand: their specific diagnosis and management. *Ergonomics*, **36**, 871–880

Stevenson, M. (1987) *Readings in RSI: The Ergonomics Approach to Repetition Strain Injuries*, New South Wales University Press, Sydney

Chapter 13

Costing

Kate S. Crocker

Introduction

A costing evaluation is a matter of calculating expected costs, estimating potential benefits and determining if benefits outweigh costs. This evaluation should be applied to occupational health physiotherapy, because in a climate of financial restraint all company departments will have their costs carefully scrutinized.

Companies may consider initiating an occupational physiotherapy service. What evidence is there to support this decision? It has been recognized that most healthcare therapies are unproven in terms of effectiveness, let alone cost effectiveness (Cochrane, 1972) and this has led to an increasing demand for literature that analyses and justifies the cost of occupational health services and prevention programmes (Moore and Hoover, 1974; Golaszewski et al., 1992). However, no such information specifically related to occupational health physiotherapy is available.

According to Maynard (1990) the following questions should be asked in all economic evaluations:

1. Are the research question and trial design clearly identified and feasible?
2. Are both the experimental and control (comparator) arms of the trial well described?
3. Are all relevant costs identified and quantified?

4. Are all the relevant effects (outcomes measured in terms of enhancements in the length and quality of life) of the competing therapies identified, quantified and valued?
5. Is the sample appropriate and sufficient in size to ensure statistical power for costs and effects?
6. Are marginal (incremental) costs and effects identified?
7. Are costs and effects discounted (to take into account time preference) appropriately?
8. Are the results subjected to a sensitivity analysis?

This calibre of economic evaluation has not been applied to occupational health physiotherapy. Physiotherapists working in this field are convinced they are cost effective. From the author's experience many company employees using the service endorse this view, but unless it is proven with accepted methodology the position of the occupational health physiotherapist may not withstand critical scrutiny and is therefore vulnerable.

This is an attempt to address some of the evaluation points. The question for discussion is:

Is it beneficial for an employer to provide an occupational physiotherapy service for employees?

First, is there a requirement for physiotherapy in the working population? This group is often physically active with high expectations of health and fitness. Some occupations require an optimum level of fitness, e.g. Fire, Police and Ambulance services. Physiotherapy is frequently used to treat injuries that occur whilst maintaining this high level of fitness.

The older age group may suffer from diseases of the ageing process. Some of the symptoms of these conditions can often be relieved by physiotherapy treatments.

In the 1991 financial year 1 736 500 initial contacts for NHS outpatient physiotherapy treatments were made in England in the 16–64-year age group (Korner Report, 1993).

The answer to the question. 'Is there a requirement?' would seem to be 'yes.' To decide whether it is beneficial for employers to meet the cost of this service for their employees, economic evaluation must be made.

The next step in answering the discussion question requires that the following alternative options for addressing this need are described and compared.

Description of the options

Option 1: Provide an occupational health physiotherapy service. Occupational physiotherapy is described by the Association of Chartered Physiotherapists in Occupational Health as follows:

> 'Chartered physiotherapists work in industry to treat injured workers, give advice to prevent further injury and help to speed recovery. Many physiotherapists in occupational health have undertaken specialised training in ergonomics to allow them to study work practices and advise on ways to prevent injury at work and promote good health. Together with other health professionals in industry they work for the benefit of employees' (Chartered Society of Physiotherapy, 1992a)

Option 2: Provide company medical insurance allowing access to private physiotherapy clinics.

Option 3: Do nothing based upon the assumption what all employees needing physiotherapy treatment will go to the NHS physiotherapy clinics. The Chartered Society of Physiotherapy defines physiotherapy as provided by the NHS or private practitioner as follows:

> '. . . the treatment of injury and disease by enhancing the body's own natural healing mechanisms. Physiotherapy is an holistic approach to healthcare including consideration of lifestyle work and leisure. Chartered physiotherapists assess, treat, teach, and advise patients'.

The treatment takes place at local hospitals or private clinics (Chartered Society of Physiotherapy, 1992b).

The definitions above illustrate the dual role of the occupational health, NHS and private practice physiotherapist.

All provide a treatment and advisory service. To assess benefit, both treatment and advisory functions must be compared with each alternative option. There are several methods that can be used to assess costs and benefits.

Methods of comparison

Cost–benefit analysis

Cost–benefit analysis (Williams, 1974) implies services should be provided only if the benefits outweigh the costs. It makes the assumptions that:

1. It is possible to separate one service from another in a sensible way.
2. There is a possibility of choice between the services.
3. It is possible to estimate the outcomes associated with each alternative service.
4. It is possible to value these outcomes.
5. It is possible to estimate the cost of providing each service.
6. These costs and benefits can be weighed against each other.
7. We should cease providing those services whose costs outweigh benefits.

When evaluating the physiotherapy treatment role the cost–benefit analysis compares the costs and benefits of providing option 1 (providing an occupational health physiotherapy service) with options 2 or 3 (not providing the service).
    Option 1 costs:

1. Physiotherapist's salary
2. Capital expenditure (discounted at 20%)
3. Facility – space rental plus utilities
4. Employee lost time.

Option 2 costs:

1. Employee lost time, taking into account travelling time
2. Insurance premium.

Option 3 costs employee lost time, taking into account travelling and hospital waiting time.

To prove the cost benefit of occupational health physiotherapy treatment service the cost of option 2 or 3 must be greater than the cost of option 1.

The application of cost–benefit analysis can be applied to the 1991 occupational health physiotherapy department statistics of a company with 1000 employees: this is demonstrated in Table 13.1. There can be many limitations with this method of analysis. In general no account is taken of:

1. Time lost for GP visit to arrange referral to physiotherapist.
2. Waiting list time for NHS physiotherapy, which can be up to 6 weeks in some areas; this may lead to sickness absence and/or impaired performance.
3. Increased treatment time required when treating acute versus chronic conditions (i.e. delay in treatment).
4. Litigation.

Cost-effectiveness analysis

This analysis is often used to assess healthcare situations. It evaluates costs against secondary monetary effects. It takes into account sickness absence statistics, injury and accident rate, compensation claims and productivity, all of which are relevant to the employer. This method is therefore more appropriate when considering the advisory role of each physiotherapy option.

The physiotherapy advisory function can be evaluated using back problems as an example. Work-associated back problems are recognized as a major occupational health problem (Pheasant, 1991): 68 million working days were lost due to back pain in Great Britain in 1991. This represents an enormous cost to industry. According to the statistics from

Table 13.1 Application of cost–benefit analysis in 1991 occupational health physiotherapy department statistics of a company with 1000 employees

Cost element	Option	
	1. Occupational health physiotherapy	2 or 3. NHS or private physiotherapy*
Salary	£18.0K	–
Facility†	£13.5K	–
Cost apportioned to treatment time only (against prevention)	£15.75K	–
Total attendances at physiotherapy department	1800 h	1800 h (assumed)
Calculated extra time (travelling and waiting 2 h per visit)	–	3600 h
Extra cost at £19/h‡ Attendance at NHS or private physiotherapy		
100%		£68.0K
50%		£34.2K
15%§		£10.26K
Total compared	£15.75K	£68.4K
		£34.2K
		£10.26K

* NHS and private options were taken as equivalent. The company did not provide medical insurance therefore the costs incurred relate to employee lost time.
† Facility calculation (based on a company policy) equals 75% salary; this includes capital items discounted at 20%.
‡ £19 per hour was used as a standard unit for lost time and output.
§ 15% was taken as the lowest figure in the sensitivity analysis. This was the percentage actually referred to the occupational health physiotherapy department by the local hospitals or GPs.

the National Back Pain Association (1990–91), lost production alone costs approximately £3bn each year.

An accepted approach to alleviating this problem is the *back school* (Zachrisson–Forsell, 1980). Back schools can be provided by occupational health physiotherapists, NHS or private practice physiotherapists; these are compared below.

Back school provided by occupational health physiotherapist

1. Back schools are tailored to a particular workforce.
2. Ergonomic advice is given related directly to the working environment.
3. Preventive back school can be run for non-sufferers of back pain, i.e. healthy workers.

Back school provided by NHS or private clinic

1. These back schools have no knowledge of the working environment.
2. Ergonomic advice is likely to be of a generalized nature.
3. Back schools will be reactive for workers with back pain.

The model in Figure 13.1 can be used to illustrate the benefit of occupational health physiotherapy compared to the NHS or private options.

This model shows that work-associated back problems are a result of a mismatch between the back stress demands of work and the individual's back stress capabilities. Intervention aimed at reducing work-associated back problems should match the demands of work with people's character-

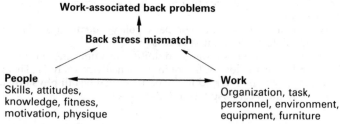

Fig. 13.1 Ergonomic model of work-associated back problems.

istics. The back stress demands of work are due to task, organizational, environmental, personnel, furniture and equipment factors. The capabilities of people to tolerate back stress are determined by their skills, knowledge, fitness, physique, motivation and attitude (Straker, 1990).

The occupational health physiotherapist is familiar with the back stress demands of work and therefore will be in a position to match these with the personal characteristics. The NHS or private physiotherapist will be able to assess to a certain extent the personal characteristics, but will not be familiar with the work demands, therefore advice and treatment will not have the same impact on back problems that are directly work related.

Example

A study undertaken by the author (Crocker, 1991) using the occupational health back school approach resulted in a 68% reduction in sickness absence for low back pain between the years 1987 and 1990 (Figure 13.2). The strategy

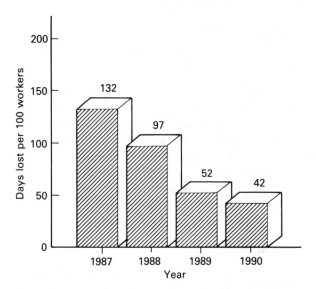

Fig. 13.2 Days lost per 100 workers as a result of low back pain.

used was to analyse sickness absence statistics to highlight problem areas and subsequently target these areas with back schools. Specific ergonomic advice was given, related directly to work undertaken by the employees.

In his book *Increasing Productivity and Profit Through Health and Safety*, Maurice Oxenburg (1991) referenced a number of case studies that illustrate beneficial ergonomic interventions. He used a comprehensive productivity model to demonstrate how employers benefit from these interventions. The productivity model is a useful tool for the occupational health physiotherapist to help prove value, and can be used to illustrate the value of the back school study mentioned above.

There are eight calculations made in the productivity model:

1. Productive hours worked for and paid for by the employer
2. Wage or salary costs
3. Employee turnover and training costs
4. Productivity shortfall (productivity losses due to absence)
5. Total costs for employment and productivity shortfall
6. Estimated health, safety and productivity benefits
7. Cost for improvements
8. Pay-back period.

This model can be used to illustrate the value of the back school study as follows. By inserting the relevant data for the study company into each step of the model, the pay-back period for the back school programme can be calculated. The worked example shown in Figure 13.3 indicates how a very short pay-back period of 4 months demonstrates conclusively the value to the company of the occupational health physiotherapy advisory back school programme.

Cost utility analysis

An alternative method for comparing the benefits of different healthcare options was developed in the 1980s (Williams and

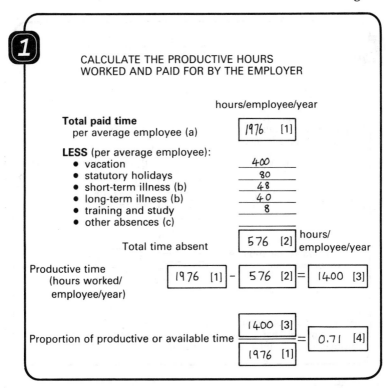

Fig. 13.3a Worked example of productivity model calculations.

Kind, 1991). This is the cost utility analysis, which measures benefits in terms of quality adjusted life years (QALYs). Competing healthcare programmes are compared in terms of their cost per QALY produced, the alternative with the lowest cost per QALY being most efficient. This is a tool that is still under development and there is speculation as to the extent of its use as well as criticism of the methodology applied. Levels of disability and distress are used to yield a QALY score. Full health (no disability or distress) is assigned a score of 1 and death a score of 0.

Various criteria have been examined when calculating quality of life ratings, and the Euroqol descriptive system (Table 13.2) attempts to provide a standard model (Williams and Kind, 1991). The application of this method in its present

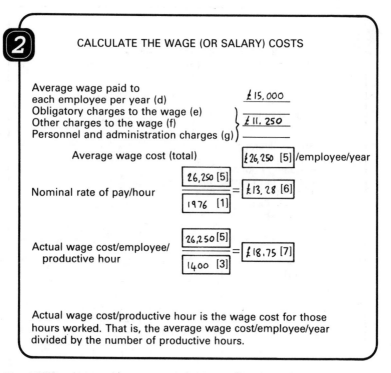

Fig. 13.3b

form has limitations when comparing the physiotherapy options available to the employer. Employees represent the major investment for a company and therefore the employer has much to gain from the workforce maintaining a '1'-coded quality of life. Not all employees will attain or sustain this rating and therefore an adaption of the cost utility model can be applied to the discussion question. The quality of life criteria of importance to the employer are mobility, ability to perform main activity and pain and discomfort.

Table 13.3 illustrates the application of cost utility analysis to option 1 (occupational health physiotherapy) compared to options 2 and 3 (private or NHS physiotherapy). By subsequently applying similar calculations to those of Oxenburg (1991), cost utility analysis can be used to illustrate the relative benefits of the physiotherapy options.

EMPLOYEE TURNOVER AND TRAINING COSTS

These are the costs for the employment of new employees and the loss of trained employees. They should be calculated separately from other administrative costs and not double counted.

2 ill-health retirements per 1000 employees

Costs to hire new employees (h):

recruitment costs
- extra administration (i)
- discussions (union/supervisor, etc.)
- advertisements, use of recruitment   £5,000
      agency, etc.)
- other

starting costs
- induction and work/safety training
      (away from the service/production area)
- training at the work station (j)   £5,000
- reduced production
- reduced quality
- other

Costs to lose trained employees:

- loss of production and quality (k)   _____

Total costs due to employee turnover | £10,000 [8] | per employee /year

The costs due to employee turnover/year [8] is converted to an additional wage cost by dividing it by the number of employees:

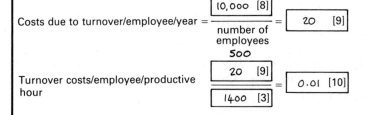

$$\text{Costs due to turnover/employee/year} = \frac{10,000 \quad [8]}{\text{number of employees} \atop 500} = \boxed{20 \quad [9]}$$

$$\text{Turnover costs/employee/productive hour} \quad \frac{20 \quad [9]}{1400 \quad [3]} = \boxed{0.01 \quad [10]}$$

Fig. 13.3c

PRODUCTIVITY SHORTFALL (PRODUCTIVITY LOSSES DUE TO ABSENCE)

Costs to replace production or services due to absence (l):

- overtime (m)   624
- over-employment (over-staffing) (n)   —
- substitution (product,
    services purchased, etc.)   —

Additional costs due to:

- lowered production   —
- reduced quality (p)   —
- loss of customers, slow delivery,
    diminished reputation, etc.   —

Total productivity losses due to absence   624   [11] /year

If you have calculated this productivity loss/year as a total company cost, it is then converted to the additional wage cost by dividing it by the number of employees:

$$\text{Productivity loss/employee/year} = \frac{[11]}{\text{number of employees}} = 624 \quad [12]$$

$$\text{Productivity loss/employee/productive hour} = \frac{624 \quad [12]}{1400 \quad [3]} = 0.45 \quad [13]$$

Fig. 13.3d

Application of the analyses

To broaden the analyses in order to answer the question for differing companies there are a number of factors that should be considered:

1. Number of employees
2. Occupational risk factors
3. Occupational fitness requirement

**TOTAL COSTS FOR EMPLOYMENT
AND PRODUCTIVITY SHORTFALL [14]**

The major costs will have been calculated in boxes [7], [10] and [13].
Add the following to obtain the total costs for employment
and productivity shortfall.

$$\boxed{18.75\ [7]} + \boxed{0.01\ [10]} + \boxed{0.45\ [13]} = \boxed{19.21\ [14]}\ \text{cost/employee/ productive hour}$$

If you have information on any of the following items, it may be
appropriate to add these too:

- extra management/supervision time
- reduced productivity from lower skills
- product damage
- plant damage
- reduced investment opportunities
- equipment downtime due to injury incidents; and
- personal losses suffered by those injured.

Fig. 13.3e

**ESTIMATED HEALTH, SAFETY AND
PRODUCTIVITY BENEFITS**

These are the benefits estimated (or
measured if made after the improvements)
to occur due to the proposed
improvements. They will include:

$$\boxed{£138\,k\ \ [15]}$$

1.32 days per worker
0.42   "   "   "
0.9 days per worker

7.2 hrs x £19.21
£138 x 1000

- reduction in absenteeism
- productivity increases
- other cost savings.

Use the costs derived in [14] for the calculation of the estimated
benefit (q). The reduction in absenteeism will only relate to the reason
for the changes made, e.g. to the work station, and not to all causes
of absenteeism. Similarly for productivity increases.
Other cost savings will relate to reductions in, e.g. supervision,
maintenance, energy usage, materials waste, etc. Care must be taken
to estimate these aspects conservatively (r).

Fig. 13.3f

COST FOR IMPROVEMENTS $£35 \text{ k}$ [16]

Obtain the estimated cost for the proposed improvements and assume that there is a single expenditure made when the improvements are introduced. The way this estimate is determined, and whether administrative and other overhead cost items are included, varies between companies (s). It is a standard item and few companies would spend money without a prior estimate.

Fig. 13.3g

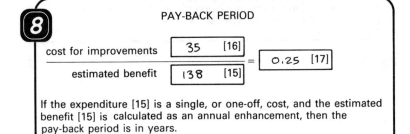

PAY-BACK PERIOD

$$\frac{\text{cost for improvements} \quad \boxed{35 \quad [16]}}{\text{estimated benefit} \quad \boxed{138 \quad [15]}} = \boxed{0.25 \quad [17]}$$

If the expenditure [15] is a single, or one-off, cost, and the estimated benefit [15] is calculated as an annual enhancement, then the pay-back period is in years.

Fig. 13.3h

4. Musculoskeletal sickness absence statistics
5. Musculoskeletal litigation
6. Accessibility of local hospital or private clinics
7. Hospital waiting list time
8. The rate at which task, equipment, etc. evolve
9. Regulatory requirements.

Having taken into consideration the above factors for an individual company, the described methods of analysis can then be applied.

Finally, occupational health physiotherapy is seen by many employees to be a 'company perk' and the benefit of this on company morale and performance should not be under-estimated.

Table 13.2   Euroqol descriptive system for rating quality of life

Mobility
1. No problems walking about
2. Unable to walk about without a stick
3. Confined to bed

Self care
1. No problems with self care
2. Unable to dress self
3. Unable to feed self

Main activity
1. Able to perform main activity (work, study, housework)
2. Unable to perform main activity

Social relationships: family and leisure activities
1. Able to pursue
2. Unable to pursue

Pain or discomfort
1. None
2. Moderate
3. Extreme

Mood: anxious or depressed
1. No
2. Yes

Conclusion

In attempting to answer the question: 'Is it beneficial for an employer to provide an occupational health physiotherapy service for employees?', this chapter has made an attempt to tackle a complex subject on which there is little published research.

Three recognized methodologies were applied to the question. These have shown that for one particular 1000-employee company with a given set of environmental and occupational factors, the answer to the question is clearly yes.

The old adage 'prevention is better than cure' from financial and moral standpoints hold true for all companies, and it is through the discussion of the preventative role that the

Table 13.3 Application of cost utility analysis to quality of life criteria of importance to the employer

	Options for employer	
Employee	Occupational health physiotherapy	NHS or private physiotherapy
Mobility		
No problems	–	–
Problems	Understanding of working environment. Advice on coping strategies whilst remaining at work	No direct insight into the working environment. May result in sickness absence
Main activity		
No problems	–	–
Problems performing main activity	Advice on adapting working practices	No specific work-related advice
Pain		
None	–	–
Moderate/severe	Immediate treatment at onset of pain	Delay in treatment

value of the occupational health physiotherapist over the NHS or private alternative is clearly shown.

References

Chartered Society of Physiotherapy (1992a) *Physiotherapy and Occupational Health*, CSP, London

Chartered Society of Physiotherapy (1992b) *Physiotherapy: Taking Care of you and your Family*, CSP, London

Cochrane, A. L. (1972) *Effectiveness and Efficiency*, Nuffield Provincial Hospitals Trust, London

Crocker, K. (1991) Reducing back pain sickness absence. *Occupational Health Review*, Oct/Nov, **33**, 9–11

Golaszewski, T., Snow, D., Lynch, W. et al. (1992) A benefit-to-cost analysis of a work-site health prevention program. *Journal of Occupational Medicine*, **34** (12)

Korner Report (1993) Form KT27, DH Statistics Division (SDLB), HMSO, London

Maynard, A. (1990) The design of future cost–benefit studies. *American Heart Journal*, **119**,

Moore, R. T. and Hoover, A. Walter (1974) NIOSH interest in the cost effectiveness of occupational health programs. *Journal of Occupational Medicine*, **16**(3), 154–155

National Back Pain Association, Annual Report 1990–91

Oxenburg, M. (1991) *Increasing Productivity and Profit Through Health and Safety*, CCH International, Bicester

Pheasant, S. (1991) *Ergonomics, Work and Health*, Macmillan, London

Straker, L. (1990) Work-associated back problems: collaborative solution. *Journal of the Society of Occupational Medicine*, **40**

Williams, A. (1974) The cost benefit approach. *British Medical Bulletin*, **30**(3), 252–255

Williams, A. and Kind, P. (1992) The present state of play about QALY's. In *Measure of Quality of Life and the Uses to Which Such Measures May Be Put* (ed. A. Hopkins), Royal College of Physicians, London

Zachrisson-Forsell, M. (1980) The Swedish back school. *Physiotherapy*, **66**(4)

Chapter 14

Research in occupational medicine

Sheila S. Kitchen

Introduction

Why do research? This question is frequently asked by both therapists and managers. If therapists are to retain and extend their status as expert practitioners, practice must be based on sound scientific principles. The evaluation of the treatment of disease by the health professions at large has generally been both inefficient and haphazard (Pocock, 1983). Physiotherapy is no execption. It is essential that this deficit be made good and that the role and practice of physiotherapy within industry is both examined and consolidated.

Research perspectives

Physiotherapy practice involves both the natural sciences, which address material phenomena, and social science, which considers the behaviour and views of individuals and groups. Research methodology must reflect these two perspectives and may be broadly divided into quantitative and qualitative forms, the latter including grounded theory research. This, however, will be considered separately in order to clarify its nature.

Quantitative research

Quantitative research methodology originated in the natural sciences and is considered by many to be primarily based on positivist philosophical principles. Bryman (1988) summarized the main principles underlying the many presentations of positivism as follows: positivism suggests that only that which is observable may be regarded as knowledge, and scientific knowledge is arrived at through the accumulation of facts gathered through such observation. Hypotheses and theories may then be derived from these observations and tested to examine their validity. Positivism highlights the great importance of objectivity in research in order to increase the reliability and validity of the observations and resultant theories.

Quantitative designs normally measure a concept which is intended to test specific hypotheses developed from underlying theories. They often examine causality and allow general implications to be deduced from specific research data. Such studies are amenable to replication and therefore testing and verification. Experimental studies, clinical trials, surveys and structured questionnaires, structured observations and the analysis of certain types of literature such as law reports may be considered as examples of such research.

Qualitative research

This form of research developed in the fields of psychology and sociology and became increasingly prominent in the early 1960s. Factors which may have effected this increase were: an increasing dissatisfaction with the use of quantitative research methods to evaluate human behaviour, beliefs and attitudes; an increase in prominence of the idea of self-reflection as described by Kuhn (1970) and the spread of ideas associated with phenomenological philosophy.

The phenomenological approach stems from the work of the philosopher Husserl and focuses on the subject and his or her understanding of the world about him/her. The approach is founded on four concepts: intentionality, description, reduction and essence. The subject consciously, or intentionally, experiences the world. This perspective is described and reduced to its essential structure. The approach focuses on the description of phenomena as described by the person, concentrating on the *essential meaning of lived experience*.

The characteristics of qualitative research are that it is descriptive, contextualized and tends to examine processes. Such methods may be more flexible than quantitative forms, concepts and theories frequently being developed as the work progresses. Verbal description, written reports and artistic expressions thus form legitimate data. Methods such as open and semistructured interviews, diaries, verbal reports and drawings may therefore be used to collect material.

Grounded theory

Grounded theory may be regarded as a form of qualitative research but is distinct from it in both its form and presuppositions and will therefore be considered separately. It arose from the study of sociology by Glaser and Strauss (1967) and shares certain common elements with qualitative research; both focus on human experience and both emphasize the importance of understanding a situation from the perspective of the subject.

Grounded theory is founded on the sociological concept of symbolic interactionism. Chenitz and Swanson (1986) stated that in grounded theory research 'the researcher needs to understand behaviour as the participants understand it, learn about their world, learn their interpretation of self in the interaction and share their definitions'. The purpose of the researcher using this approach is to *identify both the core and subsidiary processes at work in the given situation*. In grounded theory, categories are derived from data collected during fieldwork, the method allowing theory to emerge from data. New concepts and theories may be developed.

Data used in grounded theory studies are derived from a wider field than for qualitative research; they may originate from observation of social interactions, from verbal reports by both participants and non-participants, from literature and from personal experience and self-reflection. Methods used to collect data will therefore include both participant and nonparticipant observation, interviews, written reports and the literature and self-reflection.

Thus quantitative and qualitative research address different aspects of the research spectrum, qualitative research often forming a foundation from which quantitative research can continue. Both qualitative research and, more specifically, grounded theory facilitate the identification and development of new theories and frameworks of practice whilst quantitative research examines the causality and relationships.

The research process

The process required for efficient and effective research is both time-consuming and demanding and can be summarized as shown in Table 14.1. A written research protocol is usually necessary, to clarify the major aspects of study and to inform others about the aims and procedures of the study. A written research protocol is essential if the researcher is seeking funding for the study and may be necessary information for ethical committees, managers and other staff implicated in the process. Pocock (1983) provided a clear list of the components most frequently represented in a protocol.

Table 14.1 The process of research

Have an idea!
Search the literature
Develop a question
Define the purpose of the research
Design the trial
Conduct the research
Analyse the data
Draw conclusions
Publish and present the findings

Design principles and methodologies

Many research methodologies are available. A number of the most frequently used designs are discussed.

Experimental studies

Experimental studies may occur in a variety of settings and, in life science research, involve the use of body tissues, animal models or human subjects. Detailed discussion of experimental studies are provided by Pocock (1983), Silverman (1985) and Hicks (1988); both clinical trials and laboratory-based studies are considered by these authors.

The purpose of an experimental design is to examine the relationship between a number of variables which are manipulated in order to address the question under scrutiny. Experimental studies demand clear definition of the question to be asked, the variables to be examined and the procedure to be employed. The variables are defined as independent and dependent; the independent variable is manipulated by the researcher and the dependent variable is monitored for any change. All other variables are controlled as closely as possible in order that they may not interfere with the trial. Tools of measurement should be both reliable and valid. The majority of data generated from experimental studies will support the use of inferential statistics which examine relationships between the variables and the reliability of the result achieved.

Experimental trial designs vary considerably and include independent subject designs, in which the subjects are usually randomly selected and assigned to different treatment groups, matched subject designs in which matched subjects are assigned to the different treatment groups, and repeated measure designs. This last is when the same subject acts as control and subject. Such designs may be difficult to implement if time and numbers of patients are limited, but are an effective method of evaluating the efficacy of a wide variety of interventions. Thus the therapist in occupational medicine might wish to compare the therapeutic cost benefits of managing back pain through either individual or group-based care or might examine the effect of education material on the incidence of repetitive strain injury in the workplace.

Single case designs

This form of research may be regarded as a repeated measure, experimental study. Full details of the method are provided by Kazdin (1982) and Ottenbacher (1986).

The method involves a single subject who acts as his own control. The dependent variable is evaluated over a period of time to establish a stable baseline measure (A phase). Following the introduction of the independent variable, the dependent variable continues to be monitored (B phase). The intervention may then be removed and the baseline re-evaluated (ABA design) or a different intervention may be introduced and evaluated (ABC design). Many other designs have been described.

This form of research must be undertaken in a rigorous and systematic fashion: a clear question must be formulated, tools of measurement must be reliable and valid and the treatment package must be clearly defined. The analysis should be appropriate to the method and may involve visual inspection or statistical methods such as time series analysis.

The design is relatively easy to implement in routine clinical practice, and is useful when time and money are short. It allows the evaluation of subjects with unusual clinical conditions and facilitates the use of treatments which are appropriate to the individual. A single case study could, for example, provide the therapist with the means of examining the effects brought about in the presenting signs and symptoms experienced by a worker before and after changes in the design of a workstation.

There are, however, disadvantages with the method, the most important being that it is not possible to extrapolate from the findings to a larger population. Concern has also been expressed about the ethical implications of the delay in implementating treatment which occurs in the establishment of a satisfactory baseline and with the withdrawal of treatment in later phases.

Surveys

A survey has been described as a method of collecting data about large numbers of people who have been selected to represent a wider population. It involves verbal reporting of information by the subjects. Oppenheim (1992) provides detailed information about the development and use of surveys.

Two types of survey exist: the first is the descriptive, enumerative or census type of survey. Its purpose is to count and to establish facts. It will not provide information which explains or demonstrates causal relationships. Surveys may be administered to total populations, such as the National Census, or may be given to randomly selected groups. Workers in industry might be surveyed to establish the types and design of chairs they use for different purposes, the time spent each day sitting in front of a visual display unit or their views about the services provided by the physiotherapist within the workplace.

The second type of survey is analytical. This type of survey attempts to address the 'why' of a situation rather than simply the 'what' and considers the relationship between factors. Dependent and independent variables are identified and clearly defined, and the survey is designed to test these. Additional variables should be identified and controlled as far as possible. This type of survey may be used to examine the attitude, and beliefs of subjects with respect to an issue; for example, the therapist might wish to examine the attitudes of a workforce regarding the introduction of fitness training sessions, or their belief about the effects of exercise on heart disease.

A number of methodologies may be used when conducting analytical surveys; these include cross-sectional designs, before and after designs and longitudinal studies. The first makes intervention at a single point in time and relies on the sample to provide a cross-section of the appropriate population. Before and after designs examine a response prior to and following a specific intervention such as a treatment and may involve the use of a single group or a number of groups which may be the experimental, control or placebo groups. Longitudinal studies follow the group through for a period of time. Factorial designs and surveys designed to make use of regression techniques examine the inter-relationship between a number of variables, whereas matched sample designs attempt to overcome the problems associated with obtaining two groups having similar characteristics in designs which require an experimental and control group.

Questionnaires

Questionnaires have been described in different ways; they include postal questionnaires, group- or self-administered questionnaires and structured interview schedules. They may contain a variety of elements including open and closed questions, checklists, attitude scales, projective techniques and rating scales and are described more fully by Oppenheim (1992) and Streiner and Norman (1991).

The development of questionnaires demands the same rigor and attention as other tools of measurement. The question to be addressed, the aims of the study and any hypothesis to be examined should be identified. Items used may be derived from the literature relating to the area or may be developed following interviews with appropriate subjects. The validity of each item must be checked and appropriate response scales selected. The methodologies used in this context are similar to those available for analytical surveys.

McDowell and Newell (1987) and Wade (1992) provide reviews of a number of rating scales and questionnaires which are presently available for use in the assessment of health factors. The underlying concept upon which the tool is based and the known reliability and validity of each are considered. Quality of life following injury or disease, coping strategies used to manage perceived difficulties and levels of functional performance in subjects with problems such as back pain may all be examined in this way.

Observational designs

This form of research involves observing and recording information from a wide variety of sources. Whilst it is possible to argue that observation plays a part in almost all research processes, the method is most frequently used as a discrete form when studying animal and human behaviour.

Observational research demands the clear and unambiguous definition of the question to be addressed and the information to be collected. Kazdin (1982) provides information about the types of data sampling techniques which may be used in observational research. It is important that the observation procedure is conducted in a rigorous fashion. A clear statement of the objectives of the study must be developed and the observation criteria fully defined. Both the reliability and validity of the procedure must be established.

Observation may be of particular value when the subject is unable to provide the information required, when distances and times need to be accurately evaluated and to rectify received information. Observational designs are particularly useful when reported information may differ from performance; thus reports of the use and performance of lifting techniques frequently differ from actual practice. Structured observation may also assist in identifying unsatisfactory work practice and highlighting problems inherent in the design of workstations. Direct observation is inappropriate for the evaluation of opinions and attitudes and it is frequently difficult to obtain a representative sample of the behaviour being observed.

Analysis of verbal data and literature

Verbal reports, which may be derived through the use of open questions and interview techniques, and written data, such as that derived from biographies, diaries and historical record, constitute data which may be examined in a number of ways. Questionnaires and interviews conducted in the industrial setting may be analysed in this way and use may be made of diaries to record actions performed throughout the day; analysis of the contents of such information may highlight a problem which is leading to unusually high incidence of injury or high levels of absenteeism.

Content analysis (Downe – Warmboldt, 1992; Krippendorf, 1981) is perhaps the most common method used to draw systematic inferences from communications. In this method the aims and objectives of the worker must be clearly identified. Particular questions may be addressed through analysis of the literature and categories and themes are allowed to arise directly from the data. Word counts may be performed, the types of words and grammatical formulations used may be analysed and sequencing of material may be examined. Arguments presented and hypotheses developed may be identified. In this type of work, care must be taken to ensure that the data are generated in a reliable and valid fashion and that due note is taken of experimental factors, such as the form of instructions given, which can modify the verbal responses of the subject. Reliability and validity of analysis are also of importance and are usually achieved through the use of independent assessors.

Action research

Action research is concerned with identifying a problem within a specific context and then developing a local solution; it originated in education research but has spread into the caring professions. Further details are provided by McNiff (1988) and Winter (1989).

Action research is concerned with the identification of local problems, their evaluation and the implementation of local solutions. Such solutions are then evaluated and further issues identified and addressed. It is thus a cyclic process. Rigor is lent to the method by the use of reliable and valid forms of assessment and the careful implementation of change. However, this form of research remains local in its application; generalization to other populations is not possible.

Action research can be of considerable value in the industrial setting, for example handling problems may be unique to a single area within a factory or industry; action research facilitates the development and assessment of a solution which is specific to and appropriate for that location.

Grounded theory research

This form of research facilitates the development of theory from field data and has been described by Glaser and Strauss (1967) and Turner (1981). Grounded theory research could be used by the therapist in occupational medicine to extrapolate and examine the possible patterns and causes of absenteeism within a department in an industry or throughout a factory. Relationships between types of work, types of equipment used, work practices and the profile of the workforce might be identified and examined; these relationships are, however, deduced directly from the situation being evaluated and are not variables imposed on the study by the researcher.

During this process, the researcher is exposed to the field setting, collects data and develops initial categories which fit the data. Further data are sought from the field which fit within the categories. Inclusion criteria are identified for each category and a more general formulation of each is abstracted. Theoretical reflection may identify further instances which may be subsumed under each category and additional milieux in which the category may be relevant. Links between categories are noted, a hypothesis generated and conditions identified under which such conditions and connections occur. Finally, the emerging theoretical framework is related to pre-existing theoretical schemes and its validity tested through the use of other research methods.

This method is of particular value in developing new theoretical frameworks; it allows theory to emerge from data and it allows theories and categories to be developed which are meaningful to the subjects of the investigation. However, the technique may give rise to problems resulting from the mass of material which may be collected and the difficulty workers may have in freeing themselves from relevant theoretical frameworks until a relatively late stage in the process. Bryman (1988) noted that much work produced in this way up to this point in time has concentrated on categories and rarely proceeded to the development of theories.

Reliability, validity and bias

Reliability

The reliability of a tool is defined as its ability to provide a consistent and repeatable measure in a given situation. Both intra- and inter-rater reliability may be examined. Intra-rater reliability is established for a single rater over a time through the taking of repeated measures of a single parameter. Inter-rater reliability may be examined for a number of raters simultaneously examining a single situation.

Reliability is achieved through careful selection of tools, the meticulous application of the tool and attention to detail when abstracting the result. Particular care is needed when dealing with human subjects: starting positions, practice activities and instructions must be suitable and consistent.

The level of reliability demonstrated by a tool may be examined in a number of ways but is frequently expressed in terms of the coefficient of reliability; the closer this figure approximates to 1·00 the more reliable the procedure.

Validity

Validity describes the degree to which the data represent what actually happened and indicates that the tool is measuring what it purports to measure and is thus suitable for its purpose. In order to establish validity, both what is being measured and the relationship of that variable to the tool proposed should be examined.

Validity of tools may be assessed by examining face, content, concurrent, predictive or construct validity. The tool must *look* as though it addresses the area under consideration, must address all aspects of the domain under consideration, should correlate with other acceptable measures of the topic, should be able to forecast some future criterion such as daily functioning needs and should link up with theoretical assumptions about the topic. It may not, however, always be possible or necessary to examine all types of validity for every tool.

In quantitative research establishing validity is relatively straightforward; measurements of height, weight or temperature usually require little validation though they must be assessed for reliability. It would, however, be important to establish the validity of measures such as chest circumference to examine respiratory function or skin distraction of the lumbar spine to evaluate forward flexion, neither of which is clearly related to the target measurement. Establishing the validity of qualitative tools is often more complex and requires the use of a variety of techniques, which have been described by Oppenheim (1992) and Moser and Kalton (1989).

Bias

The elimination of bias is a key element in the success of a study. Bias should be guarded against through the use of rigorous design, careful training of those participating in the study and attention to detail. It may be introduced through the use of unreliable or invalid tools of measurement, through lack of experience on the part of the clinician in performing the clinical technique or assessment, through non-compliance of patients, patient withdrawals or through patient refusals to join a study. Patient and staff preferences and placebo effects may also lead to bias. A number of techniques have been developed to help reduce such biases. Double-blinding of subject and experimenter, the random selection and allocation of subjects and the careful monitoring of the reliability and validity of tools will help. Neither the ancillary care given nor the evaluation of patients should differ between treatment groups. Many additional forms of bias may arise in the use of questionnaire and measurement scales which rely on verbal self-report; the reference by Streiner and Norman (1991) deals with these in further detail.

Statistical analysis of research data

Data require examination and interpretation and it is through the appropriate use of statistical analysis that this is achieved. Both descriptive and inferential statistics may be used. The first describes the data collected and is most frequently used for descriptive surveys, questionnaires and observational data. The second allows the researcher to make inferences beyond those presented in the actual data. Most studies using this form of analysis are experimental or correlation studies. The techniques mentioned in this section are described fully in texts such as those of Pipkin (1984) and Hicks (1988).

Descriptive statistics

In descriptive statistics data may be tabulated in a variety of ways and graphs, histograms and bar charts may be used to convey information about trends and relationships in data in a clear, visual fashion.

Descriptive statistics provide information about the *nature* of typical scores and the *spread* of the scores. The first is termed measures of central tendency and includes the arithmetic mean, median and mode. Measures of dispersion give the reader some idea of the spread of the data, describing issues in terms of the range of scores, the deviation and variance of scores and, most frequently, the standard deviation.

Inferential statistics

Inferential statistics provide information beyond that which is readily available from a description of the data. Results may be inferred which relate to a wider population than that examined. The reliability of the results may be evaluated and the probability of the result occurring by chance can be assessed.

Two types of inferential statistics are available to the researcher: parametric and non-parametric. The research design used and the type of data generated will determine the form of statistical analysis to be used.

Parametric tests

A parametric test is a sensitive tool of analysis; it will highlight differences and similarities between aspects of data and determine the reliability of the result.

A number of conditions must be met if a parametric test is to be used. The data must be of an interval or ratio level. This means that the scale assumes equal intervals between the gradings. Such scales include percentages, ranges of movement, heights, weights and temperature. Additionally, the subjects for the study should be randomly selected, the data should be normally distributed and the variance in each set of results should be similar.

Non-parametric tests

A nonparametric test is a less sensitive tool of measurement than a parametric one but should be used when the data are of a nominal or ordinal nature.

Nominal scales give a name or label to a category of data. Thus, the different departments in a factory may be labelled A to G and patients attending the physiotherapy clinic may be recorded as originating from the different departments. Ordinal scales allow data to be rank ordered. Treatments may, for example, be ordered from most to least effective; appointment times may be ranked from most to least preferred. Non-parametric tools should be used in both instances.

Selection of statistical test

Selection of statistical tests depends not only on the type of data derived but also on the form of the study. The researcher must determine whether the study is designed to examine differences or similarities between groups, how many conditions, or groups of subjects, are involved and whether the subjects in the groups are the same, matched or different. Each of these factors will govern the tests used. Analysis of results must be followed by careful interpretation of the results. The relevance of the results to the subject under scrutiny and, ultimately the development of physiotherapy theory and practice, must be assessed.

Some forms of research do not make use of the above statistical methods. Qualitative research which examines verbal data and develops categories and themes is rarely allocated numerical values. Content analysis and grounded theory research are examples of research which rely on alternative methods of analysis such as frequency counts, patterning and grouping and pictorial representations.

Ethics in research

All research protocols should be assessed carefully to examine their acceptability to the subjects of the trial. No subject should be exposed to undue suffering, inconvenience, limitations or expense. This is of particular importance when considering the needs of children and those unable to answer for themselves.

The general ethical requirements for clinical research were laid out in the 'Declaration of Helsinki', produced by the World Medical Association (1960, 1975). This document clarifies the need for research to be conducted by adequately qualified practitioners, highlighting the premise that it is unethical for research to be carried out if it is badly planned and poorly executed. The issue of informed participant consent was addressed and it is noted that, in general, the subjects should be fully informed of the objectives of the work and the procedures that will take place in language which is fully intelligible to them. Each subject should understand that he or she is at liberty to refuse to participate in a study and may withdraw at any stage. All practitioners should avoid placing pressure on subjects to participate in a study and should be especially careful if the subject is in some dependent relationship with the researcher. A refusal by a person to participate in a study should not be detrimental to the treatment of that subject in any way.

In order to address these and other issues which may arise in relation to a specific study all trial protocols should be submitted to a local ethical committee for examination and approval.

The Royal Society of Medicine provides further details of the ethical issues to be considered by both researchers and ethical committees when developing and evaluating research proposals (British Medical Association, 1980).

Conclusions

Physiotherapists in all types of practice need to evaluate their current treatments and management processes; results need to be disseminated and made available to others for discussion, verification and implementation in daily practice. Physiotherapists in occupational medicine, as in other spheres, need to develop a solid theoretical basis for their practice which in turn will lead to the formulation of new professional principles and the consolidation of well-established and verified theories.

References

British Medical Association (1980) *Handbook of Medical Ethics*, BMA, London

Bryman, A. (1988) *Quantity and Quality in Social Research*, Unwin Hyman, London

Chenitz, W. and Swanson, I. (1986) *From Practice to Grounded Theory*, Addison–Wesley, California

Declaration of Helsinki (1960) World Medical Association, Geneva

Declaration of Helsinki II (1975) World Medical Association, Geneva

Downe – Warmboldt, B. (1992) Content analysis; method, application and issues. *Health Care for Women International*, **13**, 313–321

Glaser, B. G. and Strauss, A. L. (1967) *The Discovery of Grounded Theory*, Aldine, Chicago

Hicks, C. M. (1988) *Practical Research Methods for Physiotherapists*, Churchill Livingstone, London

Kazdin, A. E. (1982) *Single Case Research Designs: Methods for Clinical and Applied Settings*, Oxford University Press, Oxford

Krippendorf, K. (1981) *Content Analysis*, Sage, London

Kuhn, T. S. (1970) *The Structure of Scientific Revolutions*, 2nd edn. University of Chicago Press, Chicago

McDowell, I. and Newell, C. (1987) *Measuring Health: A Guide to Rating Scales and Questionnaires*, Oxford University Press, Oxford

McNiff, J. (1988) *Action Research: Principles and Practices*, Macmillan Education, London

Moser, C. A. and Kalton, G. (1989) *Survey Methods in Social Investigation*, Gower Publishing House, Aldershot

Oppenheim, A. N. (1992) *Questionnaire Design, Interviewing and Attitude Measurement*, Pinter Publishers, London

Ottenbacher, K. J. (1986) *Evaluating Clinical Change: Strategies for Occupational and Physical Therapists*, Williams and Wilkins, Baltimore

Pipkin, F. B. (1984) *Medical Statistics Made Easy*, Churchill Livingstone, London

Pocock, S.J. (1983) *Clinical Trials: A Practical Approach*, John Wiley, Chichester

Silverman, W. A. (1985) *Human Experimentation: A Guided Step into the Unknown*, Oxford University Press, Oxford

Streiner, D. L. and Norman, G. R. (1991) *Health Measurement Scales: A Practical Guide to Their Development and Use*, Oxford University Press, Oxford

Turner, B. A. (1981) Some practical aspects of qualitative data analysis: one way of organising the cognitive processes associated with the generation of grounded theory. *Quality and Quantity*, **15**, 225–247

Wade, D. (1992) *Measurement in Neurological Rehabilitation*, Oxford University Press, Oxford

Winter, R. (1989) *Learning from Experience: Principles and Practice in Action Research*, Falmer Press, London

Index